Notes on Prosthetic Dentistry

Dedicated to Taya, Thomas and Gill

Notes on Prosthetic Dentistry

Mervyn R. Y. Dyer, BDS, BSc, MSc, FDS, MGDS
General Practitioner
Examiner to the Royal College of Surgeons of England

Bernard J. Roberts, BDS, PhD, FDS
Formerly Senior Lecturer and Consultant,
United Medical and Dental Schools of Guy's and St Thomas' Hospitals
Formerly College Examiner to London University

WRIGHT
London   Boston   Singapore   Sydney   Toronto   Wellington

Wright
is an imprint of Butterworth Scientific

 PART OF REED INTERNATIONAL P.L.C.

First published 1989

© **Butterworth & Co. (Publishers) Ltd, 1989**

British Library Cataloguing in Publication Data

Dyer, Mervyn R. Y.
  Notes on prosthetic dentistry.
  1. Prosthetic dentistry
  I. Title   II. Roberts, Bernard, J.
  617.6'9

  ISBN 0-7236-1235-8

Library of Congress Cataloging in Publication Data applied for

Photoset by Butterworths Litho Preparation Department
Printed and bound in Great Britain by Courier International Ltd., Tiptree, Essex

Preface

For a long time we have felt the need for a prosthetic dentistry text to fill the gap between the elementary instruction manual and the large comprehensive volume. *Notes on Prosthetic Dentistry* aims to do this and is intended for students with some experience of the subject. The general dental practitioner should also find it useful for refresher and review purposes.

Since this is not a comprehensive text, we have tried to avoid contentious issues. Where differing techniques, methods or theories are discussed, sufficient references are given to stimulate the reader to obtain further information.

Suggestions, comments, notes and informed opinion will be welcomed since further editions are envisaged.

Mervyn R. Y. Dyer
Bernard J. Roberts

Acknowledgements

The authors are very grateful to those who have so willingly helped in the preparation of this book. Particular mention is due to Mr L. B. Cabot, Mr M. M. J. Shapiro and Mr R. D. Welfare, all of whom read the entire manuscript and made numerous constructive suggestions. Mr Cabot also contributed most of the contents of Chapter 18 on articulators.

Swift Data Graphics of 5–6 Clipstone Street, London W1P 7EB ably produced the illustrations.

Contents

General dental prosthetics

SECTION

General dental prosthetics

Chapter 1
Applied anatomy

In the mouth complete or partial dentures are surrounded by muscles. A knowledge of their position and action therefore enables the surgeon to construct the dentures so that they are stabilized rather than displaced. Muscles tend to destabilize the denture if they are encroached upon during contraction. Other structures such as ligaments, frena and glandular tissues should also be identified to establish their precise relation to the denture base.

The lower jaw

The anatomical structures associated with the lower denture-bearing area are (Figure 1.1):

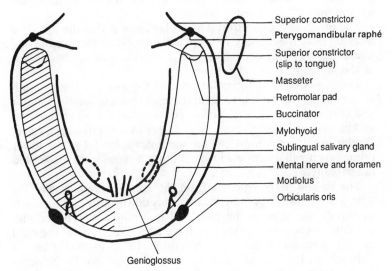

Superior constrictor
Pterygomandibular raphé
Superior constrictor (slip to tongue)
Masseter
Retromolar pad
Buccinator
Mylohyoid
Sublingual salivary gland
Mental nerve and foramen
Modiolus
Orbicularis oris

Genioglossus

Figure 1.1 Anatomical structures associated with the lower denture-bearing area

3

1. Labially and buccally:
   (a) Labial frenum;
   (b) Mentalis muscle;
   (c) Orbicularis oris;
   (d) Modiolus;
   (e) Mental nerve;
   (f) Buccinator muscle;
   (g) Masseter muscle.
2. Posteriorly:
   (a) Anterior fibres of temporalis;
   (b) Retromolar pad;
   (c) Superior constrictor (upper portion).
3. Lingually:
   (a) Mylohyoid muscle;
   (b) Sublingual salivary gland;
   (c) Genioglossus muscle;
   (d) Genial tubercle;
   (e) Lingual frenum.

The *labial frenum* is a fold of fibrous tissue in the midline between the lip and alveolus. Its width varies and it may occasionally be absent. Frena are also present buccally in the premolar region.

The *mentalis muscle* arises from the symphysis menti and is inserted *downward* into the skin of the chin. It elevates the lower lip and may lift up a lower denture.

The *orbicularis oris* forms a muscular circle within the lips. It is inserted near the midline into the labial aspect of the maxilla and mandible. Its fibres decussate (cross) with those of the buccinator at the modiolus (see below).

The *modiolus* is a muscular knot at the angles of the mouth where the dilator muscles – levator anguli oris, zygomaticus major and minor, depressor anguli oris – converge on the orbicularis oris and buccinator. This gives the appearance of the spokes of a wheel (Latin: *modiolus* = hub). As the modiolus is lateral to the lower premolars it will displace a lower denture if those teeth are set too far buccally.

The *mental nerve* emerges from the mental foramen near the apices of the lower premolars. It travels downwards and forwards to supply the skin of the chin and lower lip. In patients with extreme alveolar resorption the nerve may lie on or near the crest of the alveolar ridge and can often be palpated. Pain or paraesthesia (abnormal sensation) may be experienced if the nerve is trapped by a denture base, usually by the fitting surface.

The *buccinator* is the muscle of the cheeks. It arises from both jaws opposite the molar alveolar area and posteriorly from the pterygomandibular raphé. As the buccinator fibres run almost parallel to the denture border, they can be slightly displaced for additional retention. In this respect it is unique and it is the only muscle that can be used in this way.

The *masseter muscle* is the most powerful of the muscles which close (elevate) the mandible; in some patients it bulges towards the lower third molar. The lower denture periphery related to it should be shaped to avoid displacement when the muscle contracts.

Anterior fibres of temporalis: these are sometimes attached low down on the anterior border of the ramus as far as the attachment of the buccinator in the retromolar fossa. It is said contraction of these fibres may sometimes displace a lower denture.

The *retromolar pad* lies distal to the lower third molar and is composed of fibrous tissue and mucous glands. It is generally accepted that the underlying bone does not resorb, possibly because terminal fibres of the temporalis are inserted into it.

The *superior constrictor muscle* originates from the pterygomandibular raphe with a small extension continuing on the lingual surface of the mandible to the posterior end of the mylohyoid line.

The *mylohyoid muscle* is a thin sheet of muscle (2–3 mm supero-inferiorly) and forms the floor of the mouth. Its linear origin from the mylohyoid line of the mandible continues posteriorly to the level of the third molar.

The *sublingual salivary gland* rests on the mylohyoid muscle medial to the mandible. It is usually adjacent to the lower canine region. Its indentation is often seen on lower impressions.

The *genioglossus muscle, genial tubercle and lingual frenum:* the genioglossus arises from the superior genial tubercles on the lingual surface of the mandible. When the tongue is protruded this muscle may lift the lower denture. When the edentulous mandible is severely resorbed, the superior genial tubercle may project above the level of the alveolar ridge, and the overlying mucosa becomes traumatized by a lower denture. The lingual frenum extends from the alveolus at the base of the tongue. It is very variable in size.

Muscles limiting the extension of a lower denture

The periphery of a denture is extended as far as the surrounding musculature allows. The muscles limiting the extension of a lower denture are:

1. Anterior labial flange: orbicularis oris to lower first premolar region.
2. Buccally: buccinator.
3. Retromolar pad: buccinator and its insertion into the pterygo-mandibular raphé.
4. Lingually: the posterior extension of the lingual flange is limited by fibres from the superior constrictor, which arise from the end of the mylohyoid line and are inserted into the side of the tongue. Fibres from the palatoglossus also form a posterior limit. The depth of the lingual flange is governed by the mylohyoid.

The upper jaw

The anatomical structures associated with the upper denture-bearing area are (Figure 1.2):

1. Labially and buccally:
    (a) Labial and lateral frena;
    (b) Orbicularis oris;
    (c) Buccinator;
    (d) Coronoid process.
2. Posteriorly:
    (a) Hamular notch;
    (b) Foveae palatinae.

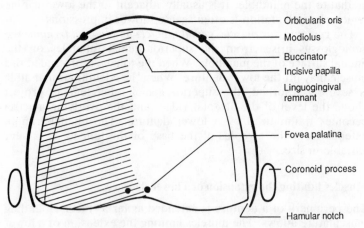

Figure 1.2 Anatomical structures associated the upper denture-bearing area

3. Palatal:
   (a) Linguogingival remnant;
   (b) Incisive papilla.

The *labial and lateral frena* are similar to the lower jaw.
Orbicularis oris and buccinator: see above.

The *coronoid process* lies lateral to the maxillary tuberosity.
When the jaw is opened it moves forward; during chewing there is
some side-to-side movement. It may sometimes impinge on the
buccal flange of a denture and cause pain or instability.

The *hamular notch* is the junction of the maxillary tuberosity
and the hamular process. The periphery of a correctly extended
complete upper denture should extend through these notches via
the area of the foveae palatinae.

The *foveae palatinae* are a pair of mucous gland duct orifices
near the midline at the junction of the hard and soft palate. These
landmarks provide a guide to the position of the posterior palatal
border of a complete upper denture.

The *remnant of the linguogingival margin* is the scar seen in
edentulous maxillae just palatal to the alveolar crest. It indicates
where the palatal gingiva used to abut against the palatal surface of
the standing teeth (see Chapter 19).

The *incisive papilla* is a small mass of fibrous tissue about 1 cm
behind the upper incisors. Its position in the edentulous mouth
indicates where the incisors and canines should be set (see Chapter
19)

Muscles limiting the extension of an upper denture

These are:

1. Anteriorly the labial flange is limited by the orbicularis oris as
   far as the first premolar region (although the levator labii
   superioris and levator angulii oris where they merge with the
   orbicularis oris may limit it in the incisor and canine regions
   respectively).
2. From about the second premolar region posteriorly, the buccal
   flange is limited by the buccinator.

The facial curtain

The orbicularis oris and buccinator muscles are draped round the
mouth to form a curtain, which is supported by the teeth and

alveoli. In edentulous patients it collapses to give the characteristic toothless look (Figure 1.3).

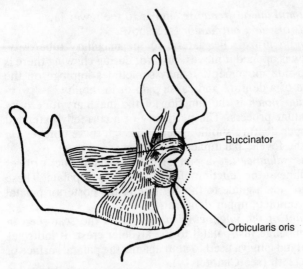

Figure 1.3 Loss of anterior teeth leading to collapse of facial curtain. Dotted line shows profile before tooth loss

Chapter 2

Causes and consequences of tooth loss: the purpose of dentures

Causes of tooth loss

Major causes of tooth loss (or absence)

1. Periodontal disease.
2. Dental caries.
3. Trauma.
4. Planned extractions.
5. Congenital absence.
6. Attrition, abrasion and erosion.

Periodontal disease is a major cause of tooth loss and the ratio of its incidence to that of dental caries is likely to increase appreciably. Since fewer teeth are being lost from caries, a greater number are retained to old age, when they are more at risk of periodontal disease.

Dental caries: the incidence of caries in the UK and, indeed, the whole of the Western world, has fallen significantly in the last decade. A recent survey reported a 50% reduction in caries in 11-year-old schoolgirls over a nine-year period.

Trauma: upper incisors are most frequently lost from accidental injury. Patients with prominent anterior teeth (Angle Class II, div. 1), especially children, are obviously most at risk.

Planned extractions for orthodontic purposes seldom lead to dentures, except where treatment has failed. Unsightly or malpositioned teeth may also require extraction.

Congenital absence: the teeth most commonly missing are the wisdom teeth, followed by the upper lateral incisors, then the lower second premolars.

Less common causes of tooth loss (or absence)

1. Anodontia – total failure of tooth development.
2. Hypodontia – partial failure of tooth development.
3. Amelogenesis imperfecta.

4. Dentinogenesis imperfecta.
5. Enamel hypoplasia.
6. Malformed or malpositioned teeth including cleft palate cases.
7. Stained teeth.
8. Resorption of teeth.
9. Cysts and neoplasms.

The cause of tooth loss should always be clearly ascertained as it may indicate the prognosis for the remaining teeth. It may also act as a guide to the patient's attitude, to the type of denture necessary, and even to the material to be used.

Consequences of partial tooth loss

The consequences of partial tooth loss include the following (Figure 2.1):

1. Drifting and tilting of adjacent teeth.
2. Rotation of teeth.
3. Over-eruption.
4. Loss of contact area.
5. Formation of food traps following (4) above.
6. Increased susceptibility to caries and periodontal disease.
7. Occlusal disruption.
8. Poor aesthetics.

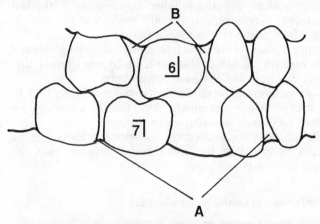

Figure 2.1 Consequences of loss of lower molar: lower adjacent teeth drift into space, leading to food packing at A; upper molar over-erupts, leading to loss of contact areas and food packing at B

9. Localized alveolar bone loss.
10. Increased likelihood of further tooth loss.
11. Fibrous replacement of upper anterior ridge.
12. See also Consequences of complete tooth loss (below).

Drifting and tilting

When a tooth is lost, anatomically unrelated teeth may be affected as well as the adjacent teeth. A single tooth or group of teeth should never be extracted without seriously considering the consequences. Where necessary, a bridge or removable denture should be provided to prevent drifting. A temporary space maintainer may be supplied while the socket heals and the treatment plan is decided.

Over-eruption

Following the loss of a tooth in the opposite arch, the over-erupted tooth is subjected to increased lateral force. Many workers believe that this accelerates periodontal breakdown if periodontal disease is already present. Furthermore, myofacial pain may develop because of the higher incidence of over-erupted teeth, spaces and locked occlusions.

Consequences of complete tooth loss

1. Alveolar resorption.
2. Anatomical structures exposed by alveolar resorption.
3. Reduced masticatory efficiency.
4. Faulty speech.
5. Changes in appearance – a prematurely aged look if dentures are not provided.
6. Psychological changes – adverse or favourable.

Alveolar resorption

When a tooth is lost the alveolar bone which formerly enclosed it tends to resorb. This is usually not obvious with only one tooth. When several are lost the reduction in alveolar height is more noticeable and the construction of stable and retentive dentures can be difficult. Some factors are known to affect resorption but in most severe cases this cannot be explained.

Factors affecting the amount of alveolar resorption
1. Local:
    (a) Provision of dentures at the time of extractions reduces total alveolar bone loss.
    (b) There is no evidence that the wearing of dentures at night or the use of porcelain teeth accelerates bone resorption.
2. General: It has never been established that general factors affect the rate or amount of alveolar bone loss. Some texts, mostly without proof, state that the following hasten bone loss:

    (a) Endocrine disorders (e.g. diabetes).
    (b) Steroid therapy.
    (c) Citamin C and D deficiency.

Resorption of the alveolus follows a definite pattern. In the maxilla the bone loss is from the buccal and labial sides of the ridge crest, resulting in an upper arch of reduced length and width. In the mandible, in addition to anterior labiobuccal loss, resorption tends to occur from the lingual aspect of the posterior portion of the alveolar ridge (Figure 2.2).

Alveolar bone is lost rapidly in the first six months following extractions and then continues slowly for many years.

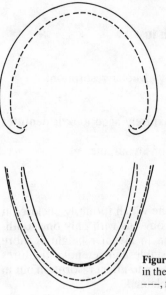

Figure 2.2 Diagram showing pattern of resorption in the maxilla and mandible: ——, original form; ---, form after years of resorption

Anatomical structures sometimes exposed by alveolar bone loss

With decrease in ridge height, anatomical structures previously not visible become prominent, and may mitigate against the success of complete dentures. These structures are:

1. The genial tubercles anteriorly on the lingual aspect of the mandibular ridge.
2. The mental tubercles – on the anterior labial aspect of the mandibular ridge.
3. The mental foramen.
4. External oblique ridge of the mandible.
5. The mylohyoid ridge.
6. The maxillary tuberosities. Resorption of bone may leave soft pendulous masses.
7. Frena. These may interfere with the ideal shape of the denture border and necessitate a large notch.
8. Incisal papilla and rugae. These soft tissue structures lie palatal to the upper incisors. After the loss of these teeth, in cases of extreme resorption the rugae may lie on the ridge crest and the papilla on the labial surface of the ridge.

Reduced masticatory efficiency

Clearly the range and type of food which a patient can eat will be reduced when he or she becomes edentulous. With a modern diet, this does not mean that malnutrition will result. Although the medical profession often relate digestive problems to lack of teeth or inadequate dentures, there is no substantive evidence for this. Some patients claim that they can eat a full range of foods with their alveolar ridges alone. It has been shown that the masticatory efficiency of complete dentures, measured as the ability to comminute certain foods in a given time, is only 25% of that of the natural dentition. The ability of partially edentulous patients to comminute their food varies, and will be somewhere between the other two figures.

Faulty speech

Although speech may be affected by total tooth loss, the range of disability varies from negligible to severe.

Changes in appearance

These include cheeks falling in, narrowing of the lips with loss of the vermilion border, and a more pronounced facial creasing. The

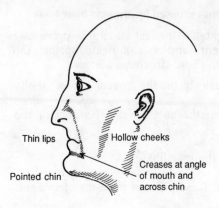

Thin lips

Hollow cheeks

Pointed chin

Creases at angle
of mouth and
across chin

Figure 2.3 Signs of overclosure
in edentulous patient

overall effect is a prematurely aged appearance with nose
approximating to chin (Figure 2.3).

Psychological changes

The patient's reaction to total tooth loss may cause psychological
changes. Age can seem to advance dramatically and some patients
cannot accept this. They frequently become problem denture
patients with the high expectation that dentures will restore their
youth.

The purpose of partial and complete dentures

The purpose of dentures is to fulfil one or several of the following:

1. Aesthetics.
2. Mastication.
3. Speech.
4. Training for future complete dentures (partial dentures only).
5. Health of the oral cavity.

Aesthetics

The loss of anterior teeth can obviously have a tremendous effect
on the patient's appearance and mental attitude. The loss of
several posterior teeth may cause a marked hollowing of the
cheeks. In addition if overclosure occurs, a protruded pointed chin
may result (Mr Punch appearance) (Figure 2.3).

Mastication

The chewing efficiency of dentures depends on many factors including the material used for construction, the buccolingual width of the posterior teeth (narrow teeth comminute food more easily) and the accuracy of the balanced articulation.

Speech

The loss of anterior teeth affects speech more than that of posteriors. The anterior teeth are the speech articulators for important consonants such as 'f', 'v', 't' and 'd'.

Training for future complete dentures

When the loss of all the remaining teeth is inevitable, the provision of a partial denture to which teeth can be added over a period of time is recommended; this will make for an easier transition to a complete prosthesis.

The health of the oral cavity

One of the aims of a partial denture is to preserve or even improve oral health by preventing tooth movement and its sequelae (see p. 10). It is important to note that any partial denture, however well made, will make oral hygiene more difficult for the patient.

Chapter 3

Jaw relationships and border paths

Errors in taking the jaw relation during the construction of complete dentures are the commonest cause of their failure.

The terminology used in describing jaw relationships can be very confusing for students. What one author means by a term may be very different to another author's usage (see Table 3.1).

Table 3.1 Jaw relationships: different terms used by authors

Term	Synonymous with
Position of maximum intercuspation (PMI)	Centric occlusion. Tooth position. Intercuspal position
Retruded contact position (RCP)	Centric relation. Ligamentous position. Hinge position
Occlusal vertical dimension (OVD)	Occlusal face height
Resting vertical dimension (RVD)	Resting face height

Jaw relationships are divided into:

1. Vertical jaw relationships, i.e. the vertical relationship between mandible and maxilla.
2. Horizontal jaw relationships, i.e the anteroposterior and lateral relationship of the mandible to maxilla.

Vertical jaw relationships

The two vertical jaw relationships important in denture construction are:

1. Rest position, measured as resting vertical dimension (RVD).
2. Occlusal vertical dimension (OVD).

The free-way space is the difference between the two.

16

Rest position

Definition: The habitual postural position of the mandible when the patient is resting comfortably in the upright position with the condyles in a neutral unstrained position in the glenoid fossae.

The physiological rest position of the mandible was defined by Wallish early in this century. Niswonger in 1938 designed the Jaw Relator and found that the average distance between rest position and occlusion in the incisor region was 3 mm. Moreover, dentures constructed with this free-way space were well tolerated. This originated the theory of Constancy of Face Height.

The rest posture of the mandible is in part a response to gravity. The physiological rest position is controlled by the proprioceptive action of the numerous muscle spindles in the jaw muscles.

Small changes in RVD occur:

1. With muscle tone changes.
2. At different times of the day.
3. With altered body posture (in the supine position RVD decreases).
4. With head position (tilting the head forwards decreases RVD).
5. If dentures are worn or not (denture wearing increases RVD).
6. With increased age, RVD increases.
7. With changes of mood (psychological stress decreases RVD).
8. Drugs, e.g. RVD increases with diazepam and decreases with caffeine.

Occlusal vertical dimension (OVD)

Definition: The occlusal vertical dimension is the vertical distance between the mandible and maxilla with the teeth in maximum intercuspation (see below).

When natural teeth meet in occlusion, the OVD is constant.

Free-way space (FWS)

Definition: The space between the maxillary and mandibular occlusal surfaces when the mandible is in its rest position.

The OVD is less than the RVD. The difference between the two measurements is the free-way space (FWS). Therefore:

RVD − OVD = FWS

The FWS in the majority of dentate patients is 2–4 mm. This should normally be followed in complete denture construction.

Horizontal jaw relationships

The horizontal jaw relationships of importance to the prosthetist are:

1. Retruded contact position (RCP).
2. Position of maximum intercuspation (PMI).
3. Muscular position.

Retruded contact position (RCP)

Definition: The jaw relationship when the condyles are in the most posterior position in the glenoid fossae at the occluding vertical dimension.

Position of maximum intercuspation (PMI)

Definition: The relationship of opposing occlusal surfaces which provides the maximum interdigitation of cusps.

In the natural dentition, provided there are sufficient numbers of opposing teeth, the position is usually self-evident. With complete dentures maximum intercuspation follows the setting up of the teeth on the denture base.

In summary, the position of maximum intercuspation (PMI) is the anteroposterior position of the lower jaw in which the teeth intercuspate maximally – whereas the RCP is the most retruded position of the mandible with the opposing teeth in contact. When the natural teeth are in occlusion RCP is 0–1.2 mm posterior to PMI.

Muscle position

If the mandible is raised from the rest position by balanced muscular activity, the point at which initial tooth contact is made is called muscle position. With natural opposing teeth muscle position should coincide with PMI. If this does not occur a potentially pathological condition exists which could cause damage to the teeth, periodontium, or temporomandibular joint.

Border movements

These are the extreme ranges of movement of the mandible. Border paths are usually visualized in the sagittal and coronal planes, i.e. viewed from the front and side (Figure 3.1).

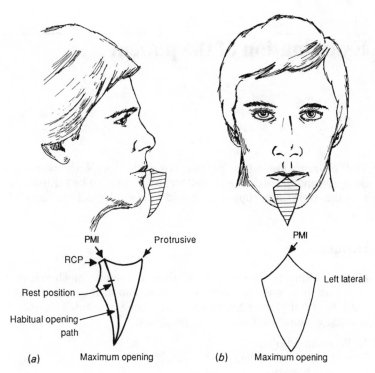

Figure 3.1 Diagram of (*a*) sagittal and (*b*) coronal border paths

To understand the sagittal border path, imagine a dot fixed to the lower incisors. Viewed from the side this dot would trace out a maximal area of movement as the jaw is protruded, then opened maximally, and finally closed along the most retruded path. The same dot viewed from the front (coronal view) would trace another border path as the mandible swings as much as possible to one side, opens to its limit, and then closes to the other side.

Chapter 4

Examination of the patient

The examination of a patient requiring complete or partial dentures enables a diagnosis and treatment plan to be formulated. It is therefore important and should follow a logical sequence.

History

History-taking is a great skill. It aims to elicit as much relevant information as possible from the patient and at the same time to put him or her at ease and in a trusting frame of mind. The history is usually considered under five headings:

1. Personal details.
2. Reason for attendance.
3. Dental history.
4. Medical history.
5. Social history.

Personal details

These are name, address, telephone number, age, family doctor (should advice be required).

Reason for attendance

A careful note should be made of the patient's complaints, requirements and expectations.

Dental history

Of particular importance are the length of time that dentures have been worn and the number of dentures constructed. A patient who has been fully or partially edentulous for only a short period and has had several dentures made, may be expecting too much from the prostheses. It is often extremely difficult to construct satisfactory dentures for these patients. At this stage of history-taking a patient's attitude and expectations are most clearly revealed.

Medical history

This can affect the provision of dentures in many ways. It is a complex matter and is discussed later in the chapter.

Social details

These include occupation (wind instrumentalists, singers, actors, models and other patients with specialized occupations may have particularly demanding requirements) and matrimonial status. It has been shown that a recently bereaved group of prosthetic patients experienced more difficulties with their dentures than a control group.

Extra-oral examination

Extra-oral examination of patient

This begins, if only subconsciously, as soon as the patient enters the surgery. Points to note include:
1. Appearance. Is the patient well groomed? Patients often have the same attitude to the appearance of their dentures as to their clothes.
2. Bearing or manner. Mild, introvert, aggressive, extrovert.
3. Appearance of teeth. Are they natural looking and of good colour?
4. Clenching or grinding habits.
5. Any obvious swelling or disproportion of face.
6. Facial colour, sweating, facial tics.
7. Palpation of submandibular and cervical lymph nodes.
8. Skeletal base relationship should be noted.
9. Temporomandibular joint (TMJ). Is there deviation on closing the mandible; clicks, crepitation or pain?

Extra-oral examination of existing dentures

1. Degree of wear.
2. Cleanliness. A patient usually cleans dentures to the same standard as the natural teeth.
3. Type of dentures: design and materials used in construction.

Intra-oral examination

This aims to ascertain the health of the patient's mouth in order to plan the construction of dentures on as sound and healthy a foundation as possible.

Examination of the partially dentate mouth

Teeth
Note the amount of caries, the quality and size of restorations, and the amount of restorative work required. This should be carefully tailored to the proposed partial denture design.

Periodontal condition
Assess the quality of oral hygiene, whether gingival bleeding is present, pocket depth and distribution, and mobility of teeth.

Occlusion
Record the number of opposing teeth in contact, and whether the occlusion is locked or the teeth can slide freely over one another. Note also the skeletal relationships and, if possible, the Angle classification.

Examination common to the partially dentate and edentulous mouths

Mucous membranes and tongue
The health of the mucous membranes and tongue should be confirmed. If many posterior teeth have been lost and not replaced by a prosthesis, the tongue may spread laterally making provision of a denture more difficult.

Temporomandibular joints
The joints should be painless and free from clicks. It is believed that a deranged occlusion will precipitate or worsen a painful joint.

Edentulous ridges
The size and shape of the edentulous ridges gives an indication of the stability and retention obtainable from the saddles. The ridges should be palpated to ascertain that there are no tender areas, which are often due to underlying bony projections.

Saliva
This fluid helps to lubricate the oral mucosa, cleanse the teeth, and prevent infection within the oral cavity. A dry mouth will make the successful wearing of dentures much more difficult.

Existing dentures

These should be examined carefully to see if there are any defects that should be corrected. If the patient is fully satisfied with his dentures, it is usually better to copy the existing design unless there is a damaging factor present such as gum-stripping.

The operator should note:

1. Complete and partial dentures
   (a) Retention, stability and extension of denture flanges.
   (b) Vertical dimension and free-way space.
   (c) Occlusion: check that when the patient occludes into RCP or PMI, the teeth meet correctly without interfering contacts.
   (d) Occlusal surface: wear facets indicate that the patient is a heavy chewer; highly polished facets indicate that the patient is a bruxist.
2. Partial dentures:
   (e) Precision of fit.
   (f) Support: are there enough effective occlusal rests, cingulum rests, or lingual plates, etc. to prevent displacement in a mucosal direction?
   (g) Clasps: efficiency.

Special tests

Radiographs

These will provide evidence of the health of the teeth and the condition of the periodontal tissues. Panoramic radiographs will give a good overall picture of the jaws and teeth, but bite-wing and periapical radiographs provide a far more detailed picture of smaller areas.

Blood and urine tests

These may be required if any systemic pathology is suspected. In such cases it is usually best to refer the patient to a physician.

Other tests

Biopsy, patch sensitivity and microbial smears or samples may occasionally be required.

Study casts

Articulated study casts provide valuable information for the construction of partial dentures. Their specific uses are:

1. To study the occlusion in detail. A lingual view of the occlusion can only be obtained from study models.
2. To study the articulation of the teeth, i.e. the sliding movement of the teeth over each other during function.
3. To study the standing teeth in detail. A decision to retain or extract over-erupted teeth can often be made more easily from study casts. The extent and nature of occlusal wear can also be determined more accurately.
4. After surveying (Chapter 8), the basis of the design can be established – principally the path of insertion which will govern the position of clasps, rests and guide planes.
5. To provide a useful visual aid when discussing treatment with the patient.
6. To construct special trays.

Medical conditions

Medical conditions may affect the wearing of dentures in different ways including:

1. Direct action on mouth, e.g. dry mouth following radiotherapy.
2. Effect on pre-prosthetic treatment, e.g. antibiotic cover for medical conditions.
3. Effect of drugs on the mouth, e.g. some antidepressants cause a dry mouth.

Note on saliva. Saliva is very important for the satisfactory wearing of complete dentures. It acts both as a lubricant due to its mucin content, and as a viscoelastic film which aids retention. Lack of saliva therefore may lead to poor retention, soreness or ulceration.

Medical conditions directly affecting the mouth

Some examples are given below. This list is not exhaustive.

1. Anaemia: soreness of the tongue and palate may occur, accompanied in severe cases by pallor and breathlessness.
2. Cerebrovascular thrombosis or haemorrhage (stroke): may lead to loss of use of the muscles of the face.
3. Arthritic disease: rheumatoid arthritis or osteoarthritis may rarely affect the temporomandibular joint.

4. Diabetes: the patient may be more susceptible to infection, and healing may be slower. The rate of bone resorption may increase.
5. Epilepsy and blackouts: the danger of fracture of a simple acrylic denture during an attack is very real.
6. Parkinson's disease: loss of muscular coordination.
7. Allergies: hypersensitivity or allergy to materials used in the construction of dentures is rarely found. Sensitivity to nickel (used in stainless steel, and some cobalt-chromium alloys) is the most likely problem to be encountered.

Medical conditions affecting pre-prosthetic treatment (especially surgery)

1. Blood dyscrasias: the resistance of the oral mucosa to trauma and oral infection may be greatly reduced.
2. Radiation therapy of the head and neck: this can lead to insufficient saliva and a readily traumatized mucosa which is slow to heal because of the poor blood supply. Furthermore the jaw bones can easily become infected following surgery.
3. Heart valve damage can occur subsequent to rheumatic fever and requires antibiotic cover for surgery. Antibiotic cover may also be needed with congenital heart disease, following heart valve surgery, and if a hip replacement prosthesis is present.

Drugs adversely affecting the provision of dentures (especially complete dentures)

1. Steroids: these suppress the inflammatory reaction and also retard healing of the mucosa after trauma. Osteoporosis (increased porosity) of the jaw bones is likely. Furthermore, long-term therapy can lead to a 'steroid crisis' during surgery if steroid cover is not provided.
2. Antidepressants: some antidepressants, especially the tri-cyclics, suppress salivary secretion. Some tranquillizers possibly also have this effect.
3. Diuretics: any drugs increasing the secretion of body fluids may lead to a dryness of the mouth, or to a change in the shape of the mucosa.
4. Immunosuppressants: these drugs are administered to trans-plant patients and for certain types of neoplasia. If traumatized the mucosa is slow to heal.
5. Anti-hypertensive drugs: some can cause a dry mouth.

Psychological aspects

The dentist–patient relationship can profoundly influence the outcome of prosthetic treatment, especially complete denture construction.

A patient's attitude is affected by the practitioner's reputation, appearance, the environment in the practice, and many more subtle features.

House (1937, unpublished) described four groups of patients, each with different attitudes to prosthetic treatment (Table 4.1):

1. Philosophical.
2. Exacting.
3. Hysterical.
4. Indifferent.

In practice the authors consider that patients seldom fit neatly into any one category but have mixtures of attitudes – often with one predominating.

Table 4.1 Effect of psychological type of patient on denture prognosis

Type of patient	Attitude	Principal characteristics	Prognosis
Philosophical	Trusting	Accept advice	Good
Exacting or critical	Doubting	Give advice to surgeon	Fair/poor
Hysterical or sceptical	Demanding	Unpleasant past experiences	Poor
Indifferent	Unconcerned	Sent by relatives	Fair

Chapter 5

Materials employed in the various stages of denture construction

This chapter provides a summary of the clinical requirements of impression materials, tissue conditioners, special trays and occlusal rims. For more detail the reader is referred to a full text on dental materials, e.g. Coombe (1986).

Properties of impression materials

Impression materials are used to record the shape of the ridges and teeth. A wide range of impression materials is available, each with differing properties and advantages. The relevant properties of an impression material are (Table 5.1):

1. Mucostatic or mucodisplacing (sometimes referred to as mucocompressive).
2. Elasticity.
3. Accuracy in thin sections.
4. Ability to be adapted and re-used for faulty impressions.
5. Mucophilic or mucophobic.

Table 5.1 Properties of impression materials

Impression material	Mucostatic	Elastic	Accurate in thin sections	Dimensional stability	High accuracy	Ability to be modified
Plaster	Yes	No	No	Good	Quite good	No
Zine oxide/ eugenol (ZnO/E)	Yes (most brands)	No	Yes	Good	No	Sometimes
Alginate	Varies	Yes	No	Fair	Quite good	No
Elastomers	Varies	Yes	Sometimes	Good	Excellent	Sometimes
Composition	No	No	No	Fair	No	Yes
Waxes	No	No	Yes	Fair	No	Yes

6. Dimensional accuracy.
7. Dimensional stability.
8. Ease of handling.
9. Cost.
10. Storage requirements.

Mucostatic or mucodisplacing

The mucoperiosteum overlying the alveolar bone and palate varies in thickness. Over the centre of the palate it is very thin. However, in several areas, for example the retromolar pad, it is far thicker and may consist of considerable amounts of fibrous tissue with numerous glands in the submucosa. Where the mucosa is thin and bound tightly to the underlying bone it is not displaceable; conversely thick mucoperiosteum can be displaced. Between the two extremes there is a range of displacement. (Note: strictly speaking, the mucosa in common with other body tissues contains a large proportion of water, which is not compressible. The term 'mucodisplacement' is therefore preferred.)

A mucostatic impression is ideally a recording of the undisplaced mucosa and is obtained with an impression material which is fluid when inserted, such as plaster. A mucodisplacing impression is a recording of the mucosa under load and is taken with a viscous material such as composition. The difference between a mucostatic and mucodisplacing impression is illustrated diagrammatically in Figure 5.1.

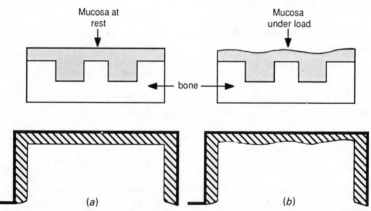

Figure 5.1 Diagrammatic illustration showing difference between (a) a mucostatic and (b) a mucodisplacing impression

There is no clear dividing line between mucostatic and mucodisplacing impression materials. For example, the consistency of alginate may vary from fluid to very stiff depending on the amount of calcium alginate and the nature of the filler.

There is some controversy as to which type of impression is best for certain clinical situations. As a guideline the authors suggest:

1. Edentulous:
   (a) Firm mucosa: either.
   (b) Flabby ridges: muscostatic impression.
   (c) Combination of firm and flabby mucosa: a combination impression using a special tray so that, for example, paste may be used over the firm mucosa and plaster in a spaced section over the flabby areas.
2. Partially edentulous: accurate reproduction of standing teeth is important but the ridges should also be considered:
   (a) Free-end saddles or large anterior saddles: mucodisplacing impression of the saddle areas so that the tissues are not displaced during function by the denture base.
   (b) Firm mucosa: either.
   (c) Flabby ridge: mucostatic impression so that fibrous tissue is not displaced.

Elasticity

Elastic impression materials reproduce undercuts accurately. This is required for:

1. Partially dentate mouths with severe undercuts.
2. Edentulous mouths with bony undercuts. Plaster, although non-elastic, can sometimes be used in these cases as it can be reassembled after fracture.

Difficulties found with elastic materials are:

1. Fracture or tearing may occur in the interdental spaces of over-erupted teeth;
2. The brand of elastic material must be carefully chosen. The tougher types – which are sometimes more accurate – may fracture plaster teeth when removing the impression material from the cast.

Accuracy in thin sections

Materials for reline impressions must be usable in thin sections, as parts of the impression are often a thin film (see Table 5.1).

Ability to be adapted if impression faulty

If a composition impression is faulty, it can often be warmed in a waterbath and re-adapted in the mouth. Stick composition can also be added – a time-saving procedure that can be particularly useful with patients who retch. Zinc oxide/eugenol paste, waxes, and some elastomeric impression materials can also be modified and re-used without completely removing the original material.

Mucophilic or mucophobic

Plaster is unique in being mucophilic, i.e. it absorbs mucus. Some patients secrete mucus excessively, especially when taking an upper impression. This leaves pools of mucus on most impression materials and produces errors on the cast. Plaster is usually more accurate in these cases. (Note: most dental surgery mouthwashes contain sodium bicarbonate which is mucolytic, i.e. it dissolves mucus. Hence rinsing with a mouthwash immediately before taking the impression will remove most of the mucus.)

Dimensional accuracy

In some procedures, particularly those which include special tooth preparations, a high degree of accuracy is required. Elastometric impression materials are particularly accurate but are much more expensive.

Dimensional stability

After taking an impression, a period of several days may elapse before it is cast. During this time materials should not distort. Alginate impression materials are most susceptible to warpage and should therefore be cast immediately. If this is not possible, as a compromise the impression should be wrapped in damp tissues and sealed in an airtight container so that water is not lost from the impression material. Composition may distort if kept in a warm environment due to stress relief.

Ease of handling

Practitioners obviously prefer materials which are easy to handle. Setting time is of particular importance. Most brands are now satisfactory in their ease of handling as manufacturers have made considerable efforts over the years to achieve this.

Storage requirements

Most impression materials now have a long shelf life but all keep better if stored in cool dry conditions.

Tissue conditioners and and functional impression materials

These are soft temporary materials applied to the fitting surface of a denture. A tissue conditioner is soft and elastic and allows inflamed and swollen tissues to recover before impressions are made.

A functional impression material undergoes plastic deformation. It is therefore viscoelastic and flows under steady pressure, but is resilient to sudden forces. The denture-bearing area and periphery are recorded during functional movements.

There is no clear dividing line between the two materials. Commercially they are usually presented as an acrylic powder, e.g. poly(ethyl methacrylate), and a liquid plasticizer, e.g. ethyl alcohol or an aromatic ester. Mixing results in a gel but it does not set chemically. The plasticizer leaches out slowly over a period of approximately one week. This leaves a hard base which should be renewed. Preformed sheets of acrylic gel which are adapted to the fitting surface of a denture are available from pharmacists and drug stores for home use. As patients often use these incorrectly, considerable long-term damage may result.

Special trays

Advantages of special trays over stock trays

1. An even thickness of impression material is produced.
2. They extend accurately into the patient's sulcus.
3. They can be modified.

Ideal special tray material

This should be:

1. Rigid.
2. Capable of modification and adjustment.
3. Stable. No distortion during use or storage.
4. Easy to fabricate.

Materials used for special trays

1. Polymeric materials.
2. Shellac.

Polymeric materials
These are usually in the form of self-cured acrylic resin containing filler. They are easy to construct and produce a rigid tray. Minor adjustments are simple but since the material is not thermoplastic, major alterations can be difficult.

Heat-cured trays are particularly rigid and strong but are more difficult, time-consuming, and expensive to construct.

Vacuum-formed plastics can also be used. These are slightly less rigid than self-cured acrylic but are more economical. The tray and impression materials should be of contrasting colours (e.g. blue tray, pink impression paste) so that defects can be readily seen. A few drops of blue vegetable dye mixed with clear polymer produce an excellent blue tray.

Shellac
This is a popular tray material as it is quick and easy to use. However, it is not as rigid as acrylic, and warpage may occur during storage or use.

Occlusal rims

These are composed of a base and a rim. Materials used for the base include:

1. Acrylic resin, self or heat-cured.
2. Shellac.
3. Wax.
4. Metal (e.g. cast cobalt-chromium palatal base plate, or skeleton framework).

In edentulous cases the base of the occlusal rim should be retentive and stable under occlusal loading, so that RCP can be recorded accurately and easily. (In partially edentulous cases retention and stability is not usually a problem, so that wax bases can be used.) Acrylic bases provide the best retention and do not flex under occlusal loads. Self-cured resins are usually used but some operators prefer heat-cured bases processed on the working models for maximum retention.

Wax is often used as it is quick and easy to handle. However, it is usually unretentive as it is not rigid and can easily become soft at mouth temperature. Rims can be constructed from wax, composition, or a plaster–pumice mix. A wide variety of waxes with different softening temperatures are available. Ideally a hard wax with a high softening temperature should be used. Composition is more dimensionally stable than wax at mouth temperature but is considerably more difficult to carve and mould. Occasionally rims are constructed of a 50:50 plaster–pumice mix. The patient can then gently grind the rims together and create the basis for a balanced articulation.

Chapter 6

Materials from which partial and complete dentures are constructed

This chapter summarizes the clinical requirements of denture base materials, clasp materials, artificial teeth and soft linings. As with the previous chapter more detail can be obtained from a dental materials textbook.

Most dentures are now made from plastic materials, usually poly(methyl methacrylate) – or metal alloys, the most common of which is cobalt-chromium. The teeth set on the denture bases are almost always acrylic; porcelain is occasionally used when wear resistance must be considered.

The choice of materials will depend upon the requirements of support, retention and aesthetics, though economic factors may have to be considered.

Denture base materials

These form the bulk of any denture and are divided into two groups:

1. Polymers.
2. Metallic materials:
   (a) Cobalt-chromium alloys.
   (b) Stainless steel.
   (c) Gold alloys.

Polymers

Acrylic resin is basically the only polymer now used as a denture base material. It has the following advantages:
1. Economy.
2. Ease of manipulation; no expensive equipment required.
3. Ease of repair and adjustment.
4. Good aesthetics.
5. Not liable to corrosion.

A denture base made from acrylic resin can be relined or rebased, repaired, or have a tooth added with the minimum of technical skill.

The appearance of acrylic is good, and the gingival appearance can be modified by the addition of small particles of red nylon. This gives the appearance of blood vessels. For patients with pigmented mucosa dark acrylic resins are also manufactured.

Although acrylic is not liable to corrosion, it may become discoloured by the action of strong bleaches, especially when these are used hot. Certain organic solvents, e.g. chloroform, will also affect the hardness and surface texture.

Other polymers have some superior properties to acrylic, e.g. nylon and polycarbonate. However these have not come into general use since they are difficult to handle and involve an injection moulding process.

Acrylic suffers from the following disadvantages:

1. Poor impact resistance.
2. Low resistance to fatigue failure.
3. Cross sections less than approximately 1.5 mm are not sufficiently strong and may fracture in use.
4. It is not suitable for constructing clasps or rests for partial dentures.

Because of poor impact resistance, the denture may break if dropped. Poor fatigue resistance results in a fracture after being used for some time. This commonly occurs along the midline of the palate of the upper denture and is due to flexing of the base during mastication. With a pronounced notch for the labial frenum the problem may be aggravated. Occlusal errors also contribute to fractures. In an attempt to improve the physical properties of an acrylic, manufacturers have modified its chemistry. Cross-linking, i.e. a type of chemical bond between polymer chains, improves acrylic hardness and impact resistance. The addition of copolymers (e.g. other polymers such as butyl methacrylate or polyisobutylene rubbers) can improve several physical properties, especially fatigue resistance. These materials are commonly known as high impact resins.

Cobalt-chromium alloys

These alloys are the most widely used materials for metal based partial dentures. Their advantages include:
1. Hardness and rigidity.
2. Corrosion resistance.

3. Strength in thin section.
4. They can relatively easily be cast and finished with special laboratory equipment.

Cobalt-chromium alloys have a modulus of elasticity approximately twice that of gold alloys, i.e. they are stiffer. This is an advantage in constructing connectors, since the same rigidity as gold can be obtained with approximately half the thickness. However, in clasps this is a disadvantage (see below). Most important of all, because of its rigidity cobalt-chromium rests can be cast to fit prepared rest seats and provide tooth support.

The disadvantages of cobalt-chromium are:

1. It is difficult to obtain a good precision fit.
2. It is difficult to repair, modify or adjust.
3. Cast clasps are not ideal.

Additions to cobalt-chromium require spot welding by skilled technicians. Bending cast cobalt-chromium is difficult: the material is brittle because of a low percentage elongation and consequently it fractures easily.

Stainless steel

Used since 1921, its current lack of popularity is due to difficulty in the manufacture of small components such as clasps and rests as an integral part of the denture base.

Stainless steel plates must be swaged on to a die, either by an hydraulic or explosive method. It has many advantages including fracture resistance, corrosion resistance, and the ability to form a very thin base.

Gold alloys

Gold is rarely used for partial denture construction because of its high cost. It can be either swaged or cast, but casting is generally the method of choice. Gold has certain advantages over cobalt-chromium, namely:

1. The casting is of higher precision due to less casting shrinkage.
2. Clasps incorporated in the framework function more efficiently (see Chapter 9).
3. Patients generally prefer gold, which appears to be more comfortable to wear. This is possibly due to its greater thermal conductivity, its lower modulus of elasticity, and lack of metallic taste which is sometimes experienced with other alloys.

Clasps

Different metals may be used to construct wrought or cast clasps as follows:

1. Cast clasps:
   (a) Cobalt-chromium.
   (b) Gold.
2. Wrought clasps:
   (a) Stainless steel wire.
   (b) Wrought gold wire.
   (c) Cobalt-chromium or nickel-chromium wire.

Cobalt-chromium clasps

These can be cast as an integral part of the framework of the denture. This is not ideal since the clasps have a high modulus of elasticity and consequently are stiff. To overcome this, the cross-sectional diameter is kept to its minimum. However, this makes the clasps more liable to permanent deformation and breakage.

Cast gold alloys

These are less stiff than cobalt-chromium with a modulus of elasticity approximately half that of the former. Consequently, they are efficient clasp materials.

Stainless steel

This has a similar modulus of elasticity to cobalt-chromium and is thus a stiff material. However this is less of a drawback than with cobalt-chromium, since it is not so brittle because of a higher percentage elongation. It can therefore be adjusted more easily.

Wrought gold alloys

These have a low modulus of elasticity. The wires are therefore not stiff and can easily be bent without breaking. Like cast gold alloys they are proved and efficient materials.

Cobalt-chromium and nickel-chromium wires

These wires have very similar physical properties to stainless steel and to each other. They are, however, slightly more brittle than stainless steel.

Artificial teeth

Artificial teeth are manufactured from acrylic resin or porcelain. Acrylic is by far the more frequently used.

Acrylic teeth

Advantages:

1. Economical.
2. Easily adjusted.
3. Bond to the denture base.
4. Can be stained for aesthetic improvement.

Disadvantage:

1. Poor abrasion resistance. Posterior teeth may wear down and so lose occlusal form.

Porcelain teeth

Advantages:

1. Hard and wear resistant.
2. Mastication is more efficient than with acrylic teeth.

Disadvantages:

1. Do not always bond well to the denture base. Chemical bonding does not occur so mechanical bonding by holes or pins is necessary.
2. Much lower thermal expansion than acrylic, thus can produce stress in the denture base.
3. Very hard to adjust for minor occlusal errors. Glaze lost with grinding.
4. May cause a clicking noise on eating if OVD is excessive or in patients wearing hearing aids.
5. Teeth may chip in use.

Attempts have been made to use porcelain upper teeth against acrylic lower teeth. In these cases, the porcelain wears away the lower acrylic teeth and an efficient masticatory surface persists for a long time.

Soft linings

Soft linings are of limited use in patients with perpetual pain or soreness of the denture-bearing area. They should not be used until all sources of irritation or trauma have been eliminated. Moreover some clinicians believe that soft linings are of no value at all. They are often used as a last resort for problem patients or for patients who insist that this feature is essential for the success of the prosthesis. However, we believe they do make denture wearing possible for a small group of 'problem patients'. Soft linings are probably most effective for reducing sudden 'impact' forces applied to the edentulous ridge, and act by absorbing some of the energy as deformation. (As an analogy punching a brick is more painful than punching a block of foam rubber.) They seem to be most effective when the patient has a thin atrophic mucosa and the underlying alveolar bone is relatively smooth.

In clinical use the following points are important:

1. The lining should be at least 2 mm thick.
2. If the denture base is weakened to accommodate the lining, stainless steel or cobalt-chromium strengtheners may be required.
3. It is best to process the denture conventionally and reline with a soft lining after the articulation has been perfected. Tracing premature contacts in dentures with a soft lining is difficult.
4. Generally soft linings are only used under lower complete dentures.

The two main groups of soft linings are the silicone type and plasticized acrylic resin. Both are made in the heat- or self-cured forms. The heat-cured forms should be used as they have better physical properties.

Silicone linings

These are rubbery materials. They are chemically resistant to food constituents, but are difficult to bond to acrylic resin denture bases and have a low rupture resistance (i.e. they tear easily). Growth of *Candida albicans* can occur on some silicone materials. They may need frequent replacement – often after less than two years.

Plasticized acrylics

These are not so soft as silicone but can be more readily bonded to acrylic resin. However, the plasticizer (commonly dibutyl phthalate) is frequently lost by leaching into the saliva. This results in hardening of the lining together with dimensional changes.

dibutyl phtalate (plasticizer)

Chapter 7

Diagnosis and integrated treatment plan

After a careful examination, the dental surgeon is able to draw up an integrated treatment plan. Where necessary this includes restoring the mouth to a healthy condition prior to the construction of dentures.

Treatment options for the partially dentate mouth

The possible options are:

1. No prosthetic treatment.
2. Fixed appliances.
3. Removable partial dentures.
4. Complete (immediate) dentures.
5. A combination of some of the above.

No prosthetic treatment

Partial dentures can be constructed for a number of reasons (see Chapter 2). If spaces are present but there is no reason or need for partial dentures, there is no point in just filling the gaps. Many elderly patients manage well with only eight teeth in each jaw, i.e. incisors, canines and first premolars. In such cases, if the prognosis for these teeth is satisfactory, dentures may not be required at all.

It should also be borne in mind that partial dentures may be detrimental to the mouth by:

(a) encouraging plaque formation;
(b) physically stripping the gingiva;
(c) predisposing to food packing; and
(d) exerting damaging forces to the standing teeth (see Chapter 13).

No prosthetic treatment is indicated in the following cases:

1. Where the denture is likely to be more harmful than beneficial.

2. In certain medical conditions such as uncontrolled epilepsy, or severe mental or physical handicap.
3. Patients of advanced biological age who have not worn dentures before.

Fixed appliances

Fixed appliances include conventional and resin-retained bridges. These are much preferred to removable dentures by most patients because:

1. They do not move during function.
2. They are less intrusive, occupying less space.
3. Psychologically, patients feel happier that the appliance is not removable.

Indications for fixed appliances include:

1. Good oral hygiene.
2. Short span to be filled.
3. Sound abutment teeth.
4. Minimal or moderate alveolar bone loss in the pontic region.
5. A gingival condition aggravated by a partial denture.

Removable partial dentures

These are indicated when:

1. There is a history of successful partial dentures.
2. The patient's oral hygiene is satisfactory.
3. There are long edentulous spaces.
4. There are unbounded edentulous areas, i.e. potential free-end saddles.
5. Severe alveolar bone loss has occurred, especially anteriorly.
6. The remaining teeth are reasonably healthy.
7. The prognosis of the remaining teeth is poor, but a 'training denture' is indicated.

Complete (immediate) dentures

These are indicated when:

1. The prognosis of the remaining teeth is poor.
2. The patient has worn partial dentures successfully.
3. The patient is young enough to adapt to the edentulous state.
4. The patient has a medical condition where the retention of dubious teeth could endanger health.

A combination of some of the above treatments

A combination may be indicated in certain patients.

Treatment plan for the partially dentate mouth

After taking the history and carrying out the examination, a treatment plan should be drawn up. This aims to create the most favourable environment for dentures. Treatment should be planned in a logical sequence:

1. Emergency treatment, i.e. relief of pain; diagnosis and treatment of serious pathology.
2. Design partial dentures (if indicated) including modification and preparation of standing teeth and crowns. Explanation to patient.
3. Periodontal treatment. Plaque control.
4. Orthodontics (rarely required).
5. Surgery (extractions, removal of roots, etc.).
6. Endodontics.
7. Conservation.
8. Prosthetics.

The above integrated treatment plan is not inflexible and, in practice, types of treatment may overlap and the order change according to circumstances.

Periodontal treatment is usually started first since it is often time-consuming. Furthermore a patient's response to treatment may require modification of the treatment plan. Surgery is performed early to allow the tissues to heal. Endodontics is performed next, since restoration of the teeth cannot be undertaken until this treatment is complete. Conservation is usually done last.

An explanation to the patient at an early stage of the treatment is most important. The surgeon should explain what he is doing, why he is doing it, and the prognosis for any planned denture.

Conservative treatment and partial dentures

Conservative treatment of teeth may aid the success of partial dentures in the following ways:

1. By providing support, e.g. rest seats in crowns and inlays.

2. By providing retention, e.g. the contouring of crowns or the placement of composite resins on appropriate enamel surfaces.
3. By creating guide planes, e.g. modification of proximal surfaces at each end of the edentulous area.

Treatment plan for the provision of complete dentures

This should be performed in the following order:

1. Treatment of urgent conditions and relief of pain.
2. Explanation to patient.
3. Treatment of systemic disease (usually by a physician).
4. Treatment of inflammatory swelling of the mucosa (tissue conditioners and adjustment of existing dentures).
5. Removal of pathological abnormalities, in most cases roots.
6. Preprosthetic surgery (see Chapter 26).
7. Construction of dentures.

An explanation to the patient indicating the prognosis for new dentures is most important. Remember that telling the patient the limitations of dentures before construction is *explanation*, after insertion is *excuse*.

The authors believe that the removal of roots is only justified in those cases where complications are likely. This is where there is either clinical or radiological evidence of infection or cyst formation, or where there is communication with the oral cavity. Routine radiographic scanning of jaws reveals a high proportion of buried roots. In one typical survey Bremner and Grant (1971) found 43% of jaws had some form of intrabony pathology, which in most cases was buried roots.

Section 2

Partial dentures

Chapter 8

Principles of surveying

The surveyor

The surveyor is an instrument designed to locate contours on teeth and associated structures.

There are many types of surveyor available. In all of these the casts are held in constant vertical relation to an instrument fixed in a vertical surveying arm (Figure 8.1). In the most common designs of surveyor the study casts are fixed on a surveying table which can be angulated in any direction and then locked in position. A vertical pillar supports a double-jointed horizontal arm with an instrument holder at its opposite end. An instrument fixed in the holder, for example a pencil lead, can be moved freely over the tooth or tissue surfaces of the casts.

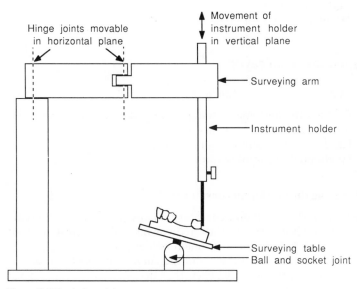

Figure 8.1 Typical model surveyor

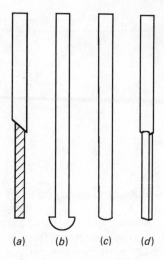

(a)   (b)   (c)   (d)

Figure 8.2 Instruments provided with a surveyor: (*a*) lead holder; (*b*) undercut gauge; (*c*) analysing rod; (*d*) trimming tool

Surveyors are usually provided with four types of accessories (Figure 8.2):

1. Analysing rod to locate maximum curvatures without marking casts.
2. Pencil lead holder.
3. Undercut gauges.
4. Trimming tool with blade edge.

Functions of surveyor

The surveyor has three functions:

1. To identify and mark the position of maximum curvature (survey line) with the pencil lead.
2. To identify the depth of an undercut.
3. To eliminate unwanted undercuts.

Identifying the maximum curvature

Identifying the maximum curvature on any tooth is done initially with the analysing rod in the surveyor and subsequently marked with a pencil held in the instrument holder (Figure 8.3). The area between the occlusal surface and the survey line is non-undercut and, similarly, the area between the survey line and the gingival margin is undercut.

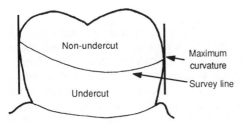

Figure 8.3 Diagram of undercut area on surveyed molar

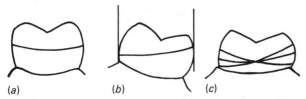

Figure 8.4 Diagram to show how survey line can change according to angulation of model. Molar (c) has been surveyed at three angulations

The survey line on a tooth is not a fixed contour and depends upon the angulation of the tooth on the surveyor table (Figure 8.4). Models may be surveyed at several angulations and so create multiple survey lines.

The depth of undercut

This is measured with an undercut gauge which consists of a rod with a horizontal plate of the required dimension at its base. Three sizes are used: 0.25 mm (10/1000″), 0.5 mm (20/1000″) and 0.75 mm (30/1000″). With the rod held against the survey line, the required gauge is moved vertically until the horizontal marker engages the tooth below the survey line (Figure 8.5). This shows the precise position of the desired undercut. If desired this can be marked with a suitable coloured pencil in contrast to the black lead.

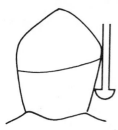

Figure 8.5 Undercut gauge in use

Elimination of unwanted undercuts

During the laboratory stage of partial denture construction, all undercuts except those to be engaged by clasps are blocked out on the master cast. The undercut is filled with plaster or wax, which is then trimmed vertically flush with the tooth surface. The trimming is done with the appropriate tool, while the cast is mounted on the surveyor table. It is important that the material filling the undercut is trimmed without scraping the plaster tooth. If the tooth is damaged the completed casting will fit the master cast but not seat in the mouth. This is because the natural tooth contours against which the casting abuts will be slightly different from those on the master cast.

Guide planes

Guide planes are essential to establish a precise path of insertion. A guide plane is a vertical portion of a tooth surface, 2–3 mm in length, over which a partial denture component can move freely. If three or four of these are present or can be created, it will only be possible to insert or remove the denture along one specific path. Guide planes are usually only effective if situated on opposite sides of the mouth or on opposite sides of the same tooth. Within certain limits the more guide planes, the more positive the path of insertion or withdrawal. An analogy to the guide plane is the accurate fit of a piston within a cylinder.

Multiple guide planes ensure that clasping is effective. It is often not realized that the mere engagement of an undercut by a clasp will not guarantee retention. For example, a clasp involving a small buccal undercut will not be retentive if the denture can be removed in a buccal direction (Figure 8.6). To ensure the efficiency of a clasp, either opposed undercuts must be engaged –

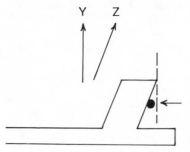

Figure 8.6 Diagrammatic section of arch. If denture can be withdrawn along direction of arrow Z, clasp is not effective. Guide planes can ensure that withdrawal is only along path Y

these are situated on opposite sides of the same tooth or on opposite sides of the arch (Figure 8.7) – or guide planes must ensure that the denture can only be removed along the path of insertion.

The stoning of interstitial surfaces of teeth adjacent to saddles can create very effective guide planes. Only about 2–3 mm of length of tooth need be stoned in most cases (Figure 8.8).

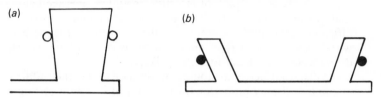

Figure 8.7 (*a*) Diagrammatic section through tooth – opposed undercuts ensure retention; (*b*) diagrammatic section through arch – opposed undercuts ensure retention

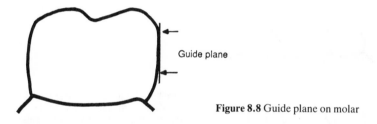

Guide plane

Figure 8.8 Guide plane on molar

Factors in choosing path of insertion

The path of insertion of a denture may be perpendicular to the occlusal plane. However, by tilting the cast on the surveyor the path of insertion may be changed at will. There is some controversy as to whether the ideal path of insertion is at right angles to the occlusal plane or angulated to it. If a right angle path is used, it is argued the denture is easier for the patient to insert and, if properly designed, is not displaced by sticky food. Those favouring an angulated path of insertion claim that the denture is more resistant to displacement by sticky foods. However, in choosing a path of insertion other factors will need to be considered:

1. The angulation of posterior abutment teeth.
2. The angulation of anterior abutment teeth.

3. The position of undercuts.
4. The dexterity of the patient.

The angulation of posterior teeth

Two situations must be considered:

1. If the proximal surfaces of a bounded saddle are both angled in the same plane, the path of insertion should be averaged along that plane (Figure 8.9). This has two advantages. First, an efficient guide plane system is utilized; second, the path of withdrawal is not at right angles to the occlusal plane making displacement by sticky foods less likely.
2. If the distal surface of an abutment tooth on a free-end saddle is angulated, it may be better for the path of insertion to follow that angulation (Figure 8.10). This makes the saddle more resistant to rotational displacement.

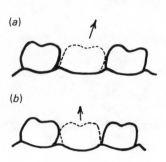

Figure 8.9 Abutment teeth angulated in same plane. Path of insertion should be along that plane (*a*), not at right angles to occlusal surface (*b*)

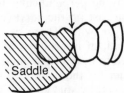

Figure 8.10 Angulated path of insertion when distal abutment is angulated

The angulation of anterior abutment teeth

The path of insertion will sometimes need to follow the angulation of anterior abutment teeth to avoid otherwise unsightly spaces (Figure 8.11).

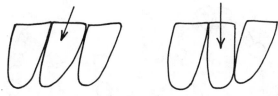

Figure 8.11 Angulated path of insertion with anterior teeth to prevent unsightly spaces

The position of undercuts

Undercuts may be created by tilting the model on the surveyor table (Figure 8.12). As pointed out previously, the engagement of undercuts is only effective if guide planes ensure a positive path of withdrawal of the denture.

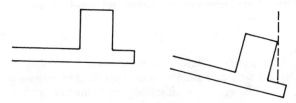

Figure 8.12 Diagrammatic section through arch. Undercut created by tipping cast

The dexterity of patients

Elderly and physically handicapped patients can find inserting dentures with sophisticated guide planes difficult or impossible.

Classifications

Various classifications of partial dentures have been formulated. Possibly their greatest use today is in simplifying descriptions. Thus 'Kennedy I' is easier to say than 'bilateral free-end saddle'.

Kennedy classification

This is the most commonly used classification and relates to the position and number of saddles. It was originally based on the frequency of occurrence; Kennedy class I was, at that time, the most commonly found and Kennedy class IV the least.

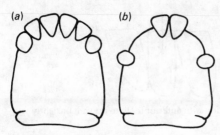

Figure 8.13 (*a*) Kennedy class I;
(*b*) Kennedy class I, modification 2

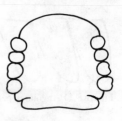

Figure 8.14
Kennedy class IV

Kennedy class I: Bilateral free-end saddle cases (Figure 8.13).
Kennedy class II: Unilateral free-end saddle.
Kennedy class III: Posterior bounded saddles, and anterior saddles not crossing the mid-line.
Kennedy class IV: Anterior saddles crossing the mid-line (Figure 8.14).

Kennedy modifications
Each extra bounded saddle is described as a modification. Thus if there were bilateral free-end saddles with two further bounded saddles in the arch, it would be described as Kennedy class I, modification 2 (Figure 8.13*b*).

There are no modifications possible in Kennedy class IV cases.

Craddock classification

This is based on the fact that a load may be tooth-borne, or tooth and mucosa-borne. The classification is:

Class I: Mucosa-borne.
Class II: Tooth-borne.
Class III: Tooth and mucosa-borne.

Chapter 9

Components of cast metal partial dentures

The components of a partial denture are usually described with reference to a single function such as retention for clasps or support for rests. In practice most components have a principle function with secondary functions which can be important. For instance, a clasp is described as a retentive component. However occlusally approaching clasps often have inflexible portions above the survey line which provide support. Similarly, occlusal rests may provide support and indirect retention.

The various components of a partial denture are listed below according to their principle function.

Saddles

Definition: That part of a partial denture which replaces lost alveolar bone, carries artificial teeth, and covers most or all of the edentulous ridge.

A saddle is nearly always constructed of acrylic resin, but where an opposing natural tooth impinges closely against the edentulous ridge, it may be constructed of metal.

Supporting components

Definition: Those parts of a partial denture which oppose forces directed towards the tissues.

Partial denture support may be tooth-borne, mucosa-borne, or a combination of the two. Only tooth-borne support will be considered here.

Tooth support is transmitted by any component of a denture which rests above the survey line. This is more effective if the component is rigid. Support is provided by:

1. Rests: occlusal usually, but also cingulum and incisal.

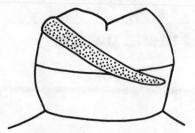

Figure 9.1 Clasp on molar viewed from side. Note large inflexible portion of clasp above survey line

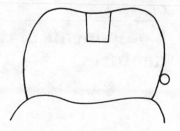

Figure 9.2 Deep rectangular rest seat preparation acting as bracing element for the clasp

2. Clasp components above the survey line (Figure 9.1).
3. Connectors which contact the tooth above the survey line, e.g. palatal plates and lingual plates.
4. Overlays and overdentures.

Functions of an occlusal rest

These may be any of the following:

1. Provide tooth-borne support.
2. Resist lateral forces – especially with a deep rest seat (Figure 9.2).
3. Restore a locally deranged occlusion.
4. Maintain precise location of clasps.
5. Provide reciprocation for a clasp (see p. 60).
6. Act as an indirect retainer (see p. 62).
7. Prevent over-eruption of unopposed teeth by resting on the occlusal surface.

Retainers

Definition: A retainer is a component which opposes displacement of a denture along its path of withdrawal.

There are four types of retainer:

1. Clasps (see below).
2. Precision attachments (see p. 61).
3. Elements of two-part dentures (see Chapter 14).
4. Flanges engaging soft tissue undercuts.

Clasps

Clasps are flexible elements of a partial denture, one part of which engages the undercut portion of a tooth. There are two main types: occlusally approaching, where the clasp approaches the undercut from an occlusal direction and gingivally approaching, where the clasp approaches the undercut from a gingival direction.

Resistance of clasps to displacement

The resistance of clasps to displacement depends on:

1. Depth of undercut engaged.
2. Material used for clasp.
3. Length of clasp arm.
4. Cross-sectional size and shape of clasp.
5. Direction of approach of clasp.
6. Position of clasp in relation to the fulcrum axis.

Depth of undercut engaged
The deeper this is, the greater the resistance to displacement.

Material used for clasp
The physical properties of the material affect the performance of the clasp. The three most important are:

1. Modulus of elasticity, i.e. stiffness.
2. Proportional limit – indicates force required to bend clasp permanently.
3. Percentage elongation – indicates amount of deformation that can occur before fracture takes place.

Length of clasp arm
The greater the length of a clasp arm, the greater its flexibility. Flexibility is proportional to the cube (third power) of clasp length. Thus, doubling the length of a clasp arm will increase its flexibility six-fold.

Cross-sectional size and shape
Increasing the diameter of a clasp decreases its flexibility. The cross-sectional shape of a clasp also affects flexibility. An example of this principle is a simple ruler. This will bend easily along its long axis in the direction of its flat surface, but will not bend along the direction of its ruling edge.

Direction of clasp approach
A gingivally approaching clasp is more resistant to displacement than an occlusal type. This is because of the angle at which the clasp tip moves over the enamel during displacement away from the tissues. The principle is similar to a fountain pen nib, which is more easily pulled than pushed over paper – the so-called trip action.

Position of clasp in relation to fulcrum axis (Figure 9.3)
A clasp pointing towards a free-end saddle is able to resist rotational displacement, whereas one pointing the other way is not able to resist this.

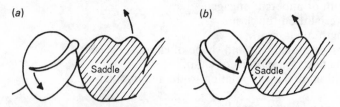

Figure 9.3 (*a*) Downward rotating clasp moves deeper into undercut; (*b*) upward rotating clasp resisted by curvature of tooth

Clinical considerations in clasp design

The actual design of clasp to be used depends on the following factors:

1. Material to be used and whether cast or wrought.
2. Depth of undercut available.
3. Position of undercut.
4. Aesthetics.

Materials to be used
The choice of material to be used is mainly based on economics and depth of undercut available (see below).

Depth of undercut available
If only a small undercut is available, an inflexible material such as cobalt-chromium is used. The ideal materials for given undercuts are shown in Table 9.1.

Position of undercut
An undercut may be high, low, diagonal or a combination of these. There are an enormous number of different clasp designs

Table 9.1 Most suitable materials for given undercuts

Undercut depth	Most suitable material
Small: 0.25 mm (10/1000″)	Cast cobalt-chromium
Medium: 0.50 mm (20/1000″)	Wrought cobalt-chromium, wrought gold, cast gold alloy or stainless steel wire
Large: 0.75 mm (30/1000″)	Wrought gold wire

available, but commonly used examples suitable for the various positions of undercut are shown in Figures 9.4, 9.5 and 9.6.

Aesthetics
This is often of vital importance anteriorly. Gingivally approaching clasps are less conspicuous than occlusally approaching. Many patients will refuse readily visible clasping.

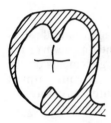

Figure 9.4 Ring clasp suitable for high survey line

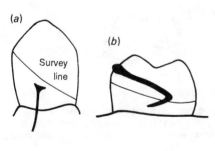

Figure 9.5 Clasps suitable for diagonal survey lines: (*a*) bar clasp (also called T-bar or roach); (*b*) recurved clasp

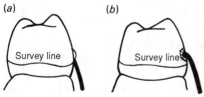

Figure 9.6 Teeth modified for low survey lines: (*a*) acid etched composite bulge; (*b*) indented inlay creating retentive pit. With sufficiently thick enamel, an inlay may not be needed

Reciprocation

When engaged in an undercut, a clasp should rest on a tooth without exerting any lateral force. However, it can be accidentally bent by the patient, e.g. when cleaning the denture. To prevent unwanted orthodontic movement, some component of the denture should be placed on the surface of the tooth opposite to the clasp. The action of a clasp should therefore be reciprocated by a non-retentive clasp arm or part of a major connector (Figure 9.7).

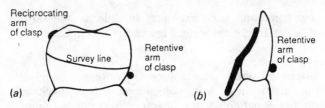

Figure 9.7 Examples of reciprocation: (*a*) interproximal view of molar showing reciprocating clasp arm; (*b*)interproximal view of canine – lingual plate acting as reciprocating element

When a denture is inserted or removed, damaging lateral forces may be applied to the teeth by the clasps as they move over the maximum curvature of the crown. Reciprocating elements on the opposite side of the teeth ensure that when the retentive arm of the clasp moves over the maximum curvature, any force is diametrically opposed at the point of application (Figure 9.8).

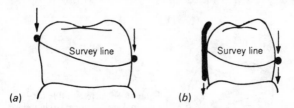

Figure 9.8 Further examples of reciprocation: (*a*) interproximal view of molar – note clasps passing survey line simultaneously; (*b*) interproximal view of premolar – note lingual plate contacts maximum curvature of tooth simultaneously with clasp

RPI clasp system

This stands for rest, plate and I bar. Instead of bracing a tooth against a buccal clasp with a lingual plate, some clinicians use the RPI system (Figure 9.9). This involves two guide planes being cut on the tooth, mesially and distally, and angled lingually towards

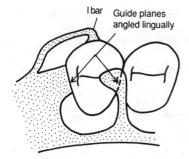

Figure 9.9 The RPI clasp system

each other. The mesial guide plane is engaged by the connector from the mesial rest; the distal guide plane is engaged by the saddle; and the tooth is clasped buccally with an I bar.

The RPI system is intended to be used on the abutment tooth adjacent to a free-end saddle.

Precision attachments

Precision attachments consist of two units – the matrix and the patrix – or colloquially, male and female; the former is usually attached to the abutment tooth and the latter to the adjacent saddle. The two units interlock to give very positive retention (Figure 9.10).

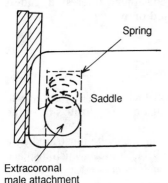

Figure 9.10 Diagram of one type of precision attachment

Advantages of precision attachments

1. Very positive retention.
2. Good aesthetic results.

3. Possible transfer of vertical and horizontal forces to abutment teeth.
4. Well tolerated by patients; their size and shape avoid intrusive elements.
5. Interlocking portions can be sprung to give a stress breaking action (see p. 66).

Disadvantages of precision attachments

1. Can involve lengthy and difficult clinical procedures.
2. Tooth preparation is usually necessary.
3. High degree of technical skill required.
4. Attachments need frequent inspection and adjustment.
5. Modifications can be difficult, or impossible.
6. Generally very expensive.

Classification of precision attachments

1. Coronal – attachment fixed to crown of tooth. This is further subdivided as to whether the male portion is attached to the abutment tooth (extracoronal) or the female portion (intracoronal).
2. Root face – attachment fixed to root-filled tooth by way of post. This is further subdivided as to whether attachment is stud type or bar type (bar supported at either end by posts entering prepared roots).

Precision attachments are a specialized subject. Interested readers are referred to the relevant texts listed on p. 202.

Indirect retainers

Definition: Those parts of a denture which provide resistance to rotation around a fulcrum axis by acting on the opposite side of the axis to the displacing force.

The principle of indirect retention can easily be illustrated by a bilateral free-end saddle case (Figure 9.11). Forces which displace the saddles away from the mucosa, such as sticky foods, cause a rotation of the denture about the rests on the premolars. In some cases the rests would lift and the saddles would rotate around the clasp tips. This causes the lingual bar to rotate forwards into the floor of the mouth. If a lingual plate was used instead, rotation would be resisted and the lingual plate would act as an indirect retainer. Rests can also be used as indirect retainers (Figure 9.12).

Large anterior saddles require indirect retention, which may be provided by rests in the posterior part of the arch (Figure 9.13). These saddles may be displaced either away from the mucosa by sticky food, or conversely towards the mucosa by incising hard food.

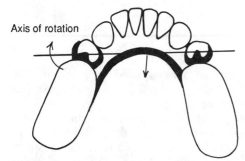

Figure 9.11 Diagram to show that if saddle of free-end denture lifts, lingual bar rotates downward into floor of mouth

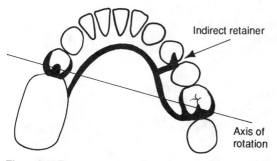

Figure 9.12 Rest seat on premolar acting as indirect retainer

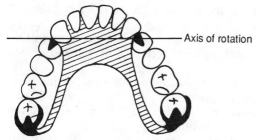

Figure 9.13 Upper anterior replacement denture. Rests and clasps on 7/7 prevent rotational displacement of saddle either towards or away from tissues

Note that in the definition above, indirect retention is provided on the *opposite* side of the fulcrum axis to the displacing force. Some clinicians believe that indirect retention can be on *either* side of the fulcrum axis. Thus clasps on the same side of the axis as the displacing force would resist rotation, and be considered as indirect retainers.

Connectors

Connectors are those parts of a denture which join the other components together. They can also fulfil other functions such as support and indirect retention.

Connectors may be classified as major or minor. Major connectors are structures which connect saddles. Minor connectors join components of the denture, such as rests and clasps, to some part of the metal framework. Connectors are classified according to their position and form:

1. Upper jaw:
    (a) Anterior, middle, or posterior palatal bars.
    (b) Any combination of the above.
    (c) Palatal plates.
    (d) Buccal or labial bars.
2. Lower jaw:
    (a) Lingual bar.
    (b) Lingual plate.
    (c) Continuous clasp.
    (d) Buccal or labial bars.

Connectors in the upper jaw (Figure 9.14)

The *anterior palatal bar* is positioned behind the incisor teeth. This connector is not usually well tolerated, as it lies in an area of tongue activity.

The *mid-palatal bar* lies on a stable non-resorbable part of the palate and is the most readily accepted of all the palatal connectors.

The *posterior palatal bar* is placed in the posterior portion of the hard palate at a variable distance from the vibrating line. Since it rests on thick glandular mucoperiosteum, it may sink during function if the denture is not sufficiently supported.

A *combination of palatal bars* is rarely necessary for cobalt-chromium frameworks, since one bar of this alloy is usually

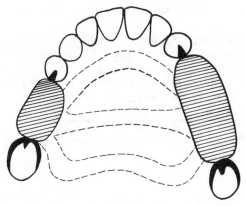

Figure 9.14 Approximate position of anterior, middle and posterior palatal bars

sufficiently rigid. Conversely the more flexible gold framework often requires multiple bars.

Palatal plates cover as much of the palate as required, and provide excellent support and strength. However they often cover the gingiva and may be less well tolerated.

Buccal and labial bars are necessary when patients are unable to tolerate any material covering the palate, or when the anterior teeth or premolars are severely retroclined.

Connectors in the lower jaw

The *lingual bar* is positioned behind the lower incisors and canines. Its upper border should lie at least 3 mm below the free gingival margin. If sufficient space is not available, an alternative connector must be used.

The *lingual plate* covers the whole or part of the lingual surface of the lower anterior teeth. It has three advantages over the lingual bar:

1. Support is obtained from the cingula of the lower teeth.
2. It is usually better tolerated.
3. It is very much easier to add a denture tooth should a tooth be later extracted.

The major disadvantage of a lingual plate is that, as it covers the gingival margin, it may predipose to periodontal disease if plaque control is poor.

Most prosthetists consider that the lingual bar and lingual plates should be rigid. This is to enable stress applied to one side of the denture to be distributed to the other. This feature is described as cross arch bracing.

The *continuous clasp* (Figure 12.1, design C) is not really a clasp as it is not retentive. It is a bar of similar thickness to a clasp which runs along the cingula of the lower anterior teeth usually in addition to a lingual bar. On the rare occasions when a lingual bar is not used it will need to be thicker. It provides effective support and does not cover the gingiva, but is often poorly tolerated.

Buccal and labial bars are occasionally useful when lower anterior teeth and premolars have a severe lingual inclination.

Stress breakers

Definition: Any device which allows movement between saddle unit and retaining unit of a partial denture.

Significantly, the most efficient and important stress breaker is the periodontal membrane. This acts like a shock absorber in a motor vehicle suspension and therefore should not be disposed of by extracting teeth without careful consideration.

Stress breakers are component parts of a partial denture which, due to their flexibility, redistribute the force to the supporting tissues. Stress breakers are, strictly, stress *distributors*. If, for example, a force of 10 kg were applied to a partial denture, this would be borne totally by the supporting tissues and ultimately the jaw bone. The force cannot be reduced or broken, merely redistributed.

Stress breakers thus:

1. Redistribute stress; more is applied to the edentulous mucosa, less to the supporting teeth.
2. May alter the direction of the force.

Examples of stress breakers

Many designs of stress breaker have been tried over the years. They are not now popular because of their cost and the difficulty in controlling the precise distribution of stress. Two examples are given below.

Split lingual plates
These may be constructed as a single casting or made by soldering a wrought gold wire which connects both saddles to a lingual plate (Figure 9.15). In this way, when masticatory force is applied to the

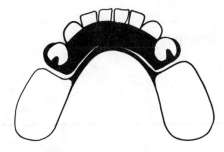

Figure 9.15 Wrought gold bar soldered to lingual plate

saddles the lingual connector flexes. More stress is therefore applied to the mucosa underlying the saddles and less to the periodontal membranes of the anterior teeth. Furthermore, since the mucosa underlying the saddles is displaceable, the saddles will sink evenly and have less tendency to tip about rigid anterior supports.

Precision attachments

These sometimes contain a stress-breaking element, usually a spring. The attachment may also be designed in such a way that movement can only occur in a precise direction. Some allow only vertical movement of the saddle, while others permit a hinge action.

Chapter 10

Partial denture design

The design of partial dentures is carried out after a thorough examination of the patient. It should be done by the clinician with the aid of surveyed study models, preferably mounted on an articulator.

Many students find the designing of partial dentures difficult. Provided the various stages in design are carried out in a logical sequence, it is not a difficult procedure.

Stages in designing dentures

The stages in the design of a cast metal denture vary among textbooks. The sequence suggested here is:

1. Select path of insertion.
2. Outline saddles.
3. Plan support.
4. Provide direct retention.
5. Provide indirect retention.
6. Join components.
7. Review.

Select path of insertion

This has been fully discussed in Chapter 8. Guide planes can be created by stoning proximal surfaces of abutment teeth in the line of the path of insertion (Figure 10.1). This produces a precise path of withdrawal which can result in an exceptionally retentive denture.

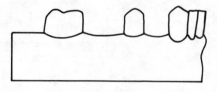

Figure 10.1 Abutment teeth stoned to create guide planes

In summary, the path of insertion is chosen in the following manner. First, the casts are placed on the surveying table so that the occlusal plane is horizontal. Usually the casts will be surveyed in this position. A note is then made of the angulation of the abutment teeth and the position of the survey lines. Most dentures will be made on models surveyed in this position. However, altering the angulation of the casts, and thus the path of insertion, may be considered in the following circumstances:

1. Where the abutment tooth on a free-end saddle case is angulated. In this case the angle of insertion may best be along the distal surface of the abutment (see p. 52).
2. Where abutment teeth on posterior bounded saddles are inclined in the same direction. The angle of insertion may best be along the common plane of angulation (see p. 52).
3. When it is considered that sticky food will displace a bounded saddle. Here the angle of insertion may best be at an angle to the occlusal plane.
4. When anterior abutments are angulated, changing the path of insertion may hide unsightly spaces (see p. 53).
5. When there is a deep undercut on one side of the arch and a shallower undercut on the other side. Sometimes a lateral tilting of the models will allow a more even distribution of undercuts.

Outline saddles

Two decisions must be taken at this stage:

1. Situation of the saddles.
2. Size of saddles.

The placement of saddles is usually a simple decision. Problems may arise if there is a small saddle space of less than half a tooth width. In such cases it may be best to leave the space unfilled.

Wherever possible, the saddle and its flanges should cover as large an area of the edentulous mucosa as possible. This distributes the load widely to the supporting tissues and helps stabilize the denture against lateral forces. With a tooth-supported saddle wide mucosal coverage is not so important. Anteriorly, a gum-fitted saddle may produce superior aesthetic results if the patient has a high lip line. This obviates the need to hide the junction between the lateral margin of a flange and the mucosa.

Plan support

Support may be:

1. Tooth-borne.
2. Mucosa-borne.
3. Tooth- and mucosa-borne.

Tooth-borne support
This is ideal because:

1. Teeth are better able to withstand occlusal loads.
2. Teeth are unlikely to move significantly during loading (alveolar mucosa may displace by 0.5 mm under load).
3. Teeth are stable, unlike the edentulous ridge which is subject to resorption.
4. Other component parts of the denture such as clasps can be more readily maintained in a precise position. If, for example, a mucosa-supported saddle sinks, the associated clasp will also sink and either become functionless or damage the adjacent gingiva.

The work of Watt *et al.* (1958) demonstrated that a patient can exert a greater clenching force on a denture saddle when it is tooth-borne rather than mucosa-borne. This is partly because the total surface area of periodontal membrane surrounding the roots of the abutment teeth is greater than that of the edentulous ridge.

Tooth-borne support is provided chiefly by occlusal rests. The choice of supporting teeth is determined by:

1. Support potential.
2. Periodontal condition.
3. Necessity for rest seat preparation.
4. Angulation of tooth.

The *support potential* of a tooth is determined by the shape and surface area of its roots. This is poor for lower incisors, upper lateral incisors, and many third molars. Canines and first and second molars provide good support. With an isolated tooth, the support potential may be reduced due to mesial and distal bone loss, whereas placing the load on a tooth in an intact part of the arch is a help, for this tooth is braced by its neighbours.

The *periodontal condition* of a tooth affects the area of periodontal membrane available for support.

The *necessity for rest seat preparation* can be judged from study models (Figure 10.2). Some patients, especially those suffering from hypersensitive dentine, dislike tooth grinding. In these cases preparation should, as far as possible, be kept to a minimum.

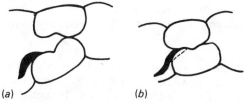

Figure 10.2 (*a*) Lower molar requiring minimal rest seat preparation; (*b*) lower molar requiring extensive rest seat preparation

Angulation of tooth. Ideally the tooth supporting a partial denture should not be angulated. Here most of the periodontal membrane bears the load, and not only half as with an angulated tooth (Figure 10.3).

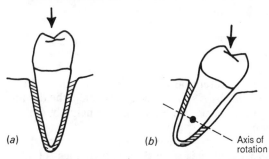

Figure 10.3 Diagram of force on teeth showing periodontal fibres under tension: (*a*) vertical tooth with all fibres under tension; (*b*) angulated tooth with about half fibres under tension

Mucosa-borne support

The mucosa is not a good supporting tissue on which to place a partial denture. A mucosa-borne partial denture may be used:

1. Where there are insufficient natural teeth to support the denture.
2. With a temporary plastic denture.
3. In the upper jaw, with a design which utilizes the stable palate, e.g. a spoon denture or the Every denture (Chapter 13).

Combined tooth and mucosa support.
This is used:

1. In free-end saddle cases.
2. With most large saddles, especially if not tooth supported at both ends.

3. With large palatal major connectors, where the stable mid-palatal area can be used for support as well as standing teeth.

In summary, tooth-borne support should be used where possible. Ideally the support should utilize healthy teeth with large root area, and be distributed evenly around the arch. In such cases four supporting components are probably sufficient.

Tooth and mucosal support will be required with free-end saddle cases, with very large saddles, and where the periodontal condition of the remaining teeth is poor.

Total mucosa-borne support is a poor compromise and should only be used where no suitable teeth are available. Mucosal borne upper dentures, however, are more satisfactory than lowers as the palate provides a stable foundation.

Retention

Clasps provide direct retention, i.e. resistance to vertical displacement. Sufficient clasps should be used to make the denture comfortably retentive. Clasps are therefore principally for the benefit of the patient.

Occlusally approaching clasps are commonly used on posterior teeth. Properly constructed, this form of clasp provides retention and support and braces the denture against lateral forces.

Gingivally approaching clasps are commonly used anteriorly because they can be made less conspicuous. Moreover, the clasp arm is usually thinner and longer than the occlusally approaching variety, and so is more flexible.

In deciding which teeth (if any) need to be clasped, the following factors should be considered:

1. The degree of retention required. Examination of the existing dentures will often reveal that the patient has learnt to wear relatively unretentive appliances. Patients wearing partial dentures for the first time usually require more retention.
2. The number of bounded saddles present. Multiple bounded saddles aid retention by forming guide planes, and providing frictional resistance to displacement by the contact between artificial teeth and natural abutment.
3. The position and depth of undercuts present.
4. The bony support of the proposed abutment teeth. Obviously teeth with poor support should only be clasped as a last resort.

5. Where possible clasps should be placed close to large saddles. This is necessary since the laws of levers show that the more remote a retainer is to a saddle, the less effective it will be.
6. The position of the lip line at rest and during function. Anterior teeth, especially canines, can often be usefully clasped. However, they will not always be tolerated by the patient if they are not fully or partially hidden by the lips.

Indirect retention

This is discussed in Chapter 9. Some form of indirect retention should be used:

1. When free-end saddles are present.
2. When there are large anterior saddles.

Any component of the metal casting on the opposite side of the fulcrum axis to the free-end saddle acts as an indirect retainer, provided it is placed above the survey line of the tooth. Commonly used indirect retainers are lingual plates, continuous clasps, cingulum rests and occlusal rests.

Similarly with anterior saddles, the indirect retainer must be placed on the opposite side of the fulcrum axis. Commonly used indirect retainers in this situation are occlusal rests and palatal plates.

Join components

Major connectors unite saddles. Minor connectors join components such as clasps and rests to the denture base. When planning connectors sufficient space must be available. Space may be created for minor connectors by tooth preparation, but major connectors have to be designed according to the features of the jaw. For example, a lingual bar requires a depth of about 8 mm from the gingival margin to the floor of the mouth. If this is not present a lingual plate will need to be used.

The type of major connector to be used may well have been chosen earlier in the design sequence, e.g. a lingual plate for tooth-borne support, or a palatal plate for indirect retention.

When choosing a major connector there are three principal considerations:

1. Is it biologically satisfactory?
2. Is it mechanically satisfactory?
3. Is it likely to be comfortable for the patient?

Review

After completing the initial design for a cast metal denture, the operator should review the design, particularly with regard to three factors:

1. Adequate lateral and anteroposterior bracing.
2. Aesthetics.
3. Simplicity of design.

Further bracing against horizontal displacement is not usually necessary, since in most cases sufficient clasps, flanges, connectors, etc. will be available to resist this displacement. A bilateral free-end saddle with flat edentulous ridges may require bracing. In such cases a lingual plate may have to be included to resist lateral displacement.

The aesthetic appearance of the denture should be considered. Many patients will not wear a denture however well designed, unless they are happy with the appearance of it.

Finally the surgeon should satisfy himself that the design is as simple as can be devised. Complex designs prejudice the remaining teeth by creating areas in which food lodges while eating, and also encourage the formation of plaque on the remaining standing teeth.

At the completion of a design the key question must be: 'Is this the most aesthetic and simple design, which will help preserve the remaining teeth, whilst replacing those which are lost?'

Chapter 11

Clinical stages in the construction of partial dentures

The clinical stages in the construction of cast metal partial dentures are:

1. Examination, diagnosis and treatment plan.
2. Primary impressions and designing dentures.
3. Preparatory treatment, e.g. periodontal and conservative treatment, etc.
4. Tooth preparation.
5. Secondary impressions.
6. Record jaw relationship.
7. Try-in metal casting.
8. Trial insertion.
9. Insertion.
10. Review.

The sequence of clinical stages does not always follow the above. For example, in cases with sufficient opposing teeth, centric occlusion can be ascertained at the primary impression stage.

Examination and diagnosis

This is fully described in Chapter 4. Information should be obtained at this stage to enable the surgeon to form a treatment plan.

Primary impressions

Primary impressions are usually taken in alginate using stock trays. Full extension of the impression is desirable, and may be obtained by modifying the stock tray with impression compound.

After the impressions have been cast, the models are surveyed and a provisional design formulated. In many cases the inter-relationship of opposing teeth can only be satisfactorily studied after the casts have been mounted on an articulator. This may need to be modified at a later date, with reference to the success of periodontal and conservative treatment.

Preparatory treatment

Clinical treatment prior to the construction of partial dentures is fully described in Chapter 7 (see p. 42).

Tooth preparation

Five types of tooth preparation may be required:

1. Occlusal rest seats.
2. Canine rest seats.
3. Grooves for clasps.
4. The creation of retentive areas.
5. Guide planes.

Occlusal rest seats

These must cover sufficient tooth area to transmit the load effectively to the tooth. They must also be sufficiently deep to allow for the strength of the rest. Figure 11.1 shows the classical shape of an occlusal rest in a premolar. The depth of the body of the rest seat preparation with the teeth in occlusion should be 1 mm, increasing to 1.5 mm in the area of the marginal ridge. Cast gold rests should be 30% thicker. The floor of the rest seat is usually saucer-shaped. Occasionally rest seats are cut deeper and squarer to produce a bracing effect.

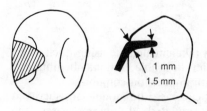

Figure 11.1 Occlusal and buccal view of ideal occlusal rest

Canine rest seats

These are best placed in teeth with pronounced cingula. The floor of the rests should extend 1 mm into the enamel and be at right angles to the long axis of the tooth. The preparation should be 2–3 mm wide (Figure 11.2).

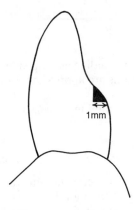

1mm

Figure 11.2 Side view of canine showing position and shape of cingulum rest

Grooves for clasps

With the teeth in occlusion there is often insufficient space to pass a clasp from the casting through to the buccal surface of a tooth (Figure 11.3). In these cases a groove about 1 mm in diameter will need to be cut.

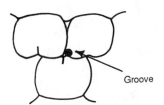

Groove

Figure 11.3 Buccal view of arch with tight occlusion. A groove may need to be cut to accommodate the clasp arm

Creating retention

Undercuts are created by cutting a dimple in the enamel with a small round bur. This should be about 0.5 mm deep and 1 mm wide – sufficient to seat either a cobalt-chromium I bar or a wrought gold wire expanded to a ball end (Figure 11.4).

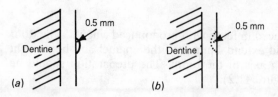

Figure 11.4 Creation of retention: (*a*) by bonding composite resin onto enamel; (*b*) by cutting dimple in enamel

A small protuberance is easily produced by bonding a composite resin on to acid-etched enamel. The dimensions are approximately the same as for a dimple.

Undercuts and dimples may also be incorporated in crowns and inlays.

Guide planes

These have been described in Chapter 8. It is often helpful to prepare these on study casts before working in the mouth. Guide planes are best prepared with a cylindrical bur and finished with polishing discs. An effective guide plane need only be 3 mm in length and width (Figure 11.5).

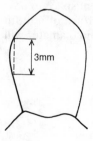

Figure 11.5 Tooth preparation for guide plane in premolar

Secondary impressions

These must not be taken until all mouth preparations are complete. Metal stock trays are often suitable and have the advantage of being rigid. Special acrylic resin trays will be required where no suitably shaped stock tray is available. However, special care must be taken in their use since perforated trays can be flexible.

Alginate is the most frequently used impression material but elastomers are required in cases with severe undercuts. To obtain a clear recording of rest seats and other fine details, it is beneficial to coat the surface of the teeth with impression material before the tray is inserted.

Recording the occlusion

Partial dentures are usually constructed to a position of maximum intercuspation and not retruded contact position (RCP) (see Chapter 3). There may be sufficient cusp to fossa contacts for maximum intercuspation to be obvious. However, if the occlusion needs to be recorded, upper or lower wax rims – or both – are used. If there are no teeth in occlusal contact, the occlusion is determined in the same way as for complete dentures and RCP is recorded.

Try-in metal casting

The metal casting is carefully examined on and off the master model, and then inserted in the mouth to assess if it fits satisfactorily. If the casting does not seat fully, it is usually possible to locate the general area of obstruction visually. The corresponding area of the fitting surface of the metal is then painted with pink stencil correcting fluid or a proprietary disclosing paste. Areas where the base shows through the disclosing material are then relieved. A particular check should be made of the following:

1. Rests correctly seated.
2. Clasps – sufficient retention but not overtight.
3. No interference with occlusion by metal components.
4. Good contact of palatal and lingual bars with the tissues.

Trial insertion

The casting with artificial teeth mounted on wax saddles is tried-in. As the metal framework had correctly fitted at the previous appointment the following features remain to be checked:

1. Aesthetics.
2. Occlusion.
3. Extension of saddles.

Insertion of denture

At this stage the main points to check are:

1. Ease of insertion of dentures.
2. Occlusion and articulation (the even contact of opposing teeth during sliding movements).
3. Extension of saddles.

Sometimes difficulty is experienced in inserting the completed denture. Disclosing waxes or pastes are then used to locate the fault. Since it has previously been shown that the metal framework is satisfactory, it should only be the acrylic which needs adjustment.

When the denture fits satisfactorily, the patient is shown how to insert and remove it without using the clasps as levers. Finally the patient is given verbal and preferably written instructions on the care of the dentures (see below).

Review

An appointment is made about a week after insertion to check that the prosthesis is satisfactory to both patient and operator.

Care of partial dentures

It is helpful to have a printed advice sheet concerning the care of partial dentures. This can be given to the patients to study at their leisure. A sample sheet is reproduced in Figure 11.6.

Comments about guidance sheet (Figure 11.6)

Some National Health patients who only pay a portion of the cost of dentures (or even none at all) do not realize how expensive they can be.

Research (Murray *et al.*, 1986) has shown that, although modern toothpastes are slightly more abrasive than special denture pastes, the total loss of acrylic over several years is negligible. Toothpaste is also readily available in most households.

The instructions diplomatically state: 'If at all possible dentures should not be worn at night'. Young patients with anterior teeth missing are unlikely to leave dentures out, whatever they are told. In such cases the oral hygiene should be beyond reproach.

Care of your partial dentures

Dentures are expensive. If you look after them well they will last longer, look better, and be more comfortable. The notes below show how to treat your dentures.

1. *If your dentures hurt* take them out and leave in water. Make an appointment to see your dentist. Wear them for 4 hours before going to your dentist so that he can see where they are rubbing.
2. *Clean* your dentures with a medium grade tooth brush or denture brush. Toothpaste is satisfactory. Whilst cleaning do not hold them by any thin wires. If you soak them in a special denture cleaner, brush and rinse them afterwards.
3. *Dentures with metal parts* should *never* be soaked in bleach.
4. *Keep your dentures in water* when not using them. This stops warping of the plastic.
5. *At night.* If at all possible dentures should not be worn at night as this encourages decay and gum trouble. If worn at night the dentures and natural teeth must be very clean.
6. *Thin metal parts* of the denture should not be used to help remove it from your mouth.
7. *Check up.* You should return to your dentist in .... months to check your dentures are still fitting properly. Then every year for a routine check of the dentures.

Figure 11.6 Sample sheet: Care of your partial dentures

The number of months before the patient's first review is entered in the space provided. For most partial denture patients this will be in six months time. At this check-up the dental surgeon will confirm that resorption, particularly in free-end saddle cases, has not caused any tipping movements. He should also check that the dentures do not predispose to plaque formation on the standing teeth, making them liable to caries or periodontal disease. Wearing any partial denture, however well made, makes oral hygiene more difficult and necessitates extra attention to this detail.

Chapter 12

Design examples of partial dentures

Many partial denture textbooks give pages of designs which have been blindly copied by generations of students who choose the example which most closely resembles the case in hand. There is no one design of partial denture that is suitable for a certain pattern of missing teeth. Many factors will affect the final design, especially:

1. The periodontal condition.
2. The position and depth of undercuts.
3. The angulation of abutment teeth.
4. The size and shape of the edentulous ridge.
5. The denture-wearing history of the patient.

The design examples given below are in no way meant to be comprehensive but are intended to indicate the thought processes involved in designing a denture.

Lower bilateral free-end saddle (Figure 12.1)

Design A

No denture. For many years this elderly patient had only her upper and lower first premolars, canines and incisors standing. Her teeth and periodontium were healthy and she was able to chew satisfactorily. It was felt that the provision of dentures would be of no benefit.

Design B

A lingual bar was chosen because of the patient's poor oral hygiene with gingival pockets around the anterior teeth. Rests were placed on all the lower premolars to obtain good support; the distal rest on the lower first premolar provided a little indirect retention. The second premolar carried a simple cast occlusally approaching clasp, necessitated by a shallow undercut. (Gingivally

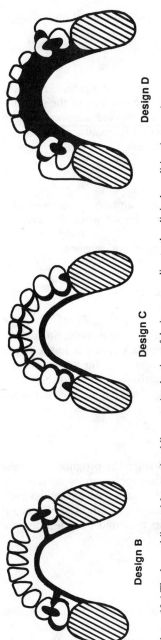

Figure 12.1 The lower bilateral free-end saddle case. A selection of designs according to the clinical condition (see text)

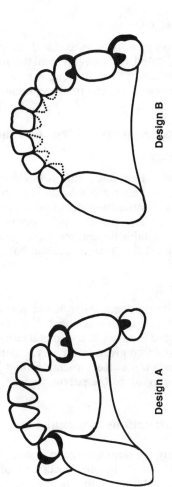

Figure 12.2 The upper unilateral free-end saddle. Two designs formulated according to the clinical condition (see text)

approaching clasps are not usually suitable for small undercuts of
0.25 mm or less.)

Design C

This patient was provided with a simple denture. Since the
periodontal condition was poor with some mobility of the standing
teeth, a continuous clasp was able to provide support without
covering the gingiva. No clasping was used because the patient's
previous satisfactory denture was claspless.

Design D

A lingual plate was used to provide support. This was also
indicated because the patient had previously worn this type of
connector. Oral hygiene was good. Gingivally approaching clasps
were used on the first premolars for aesthetic reasons.

Upper unilateral free-end saddle (Figure 12.2)

Design A

The patient had a mid-palatal bar since a mid or posterior palatal
bar is the most comfortable form of major connector in the upper
jaw. Furthermore this mid-palatal strap covers the stable portion
of the hard palate which does not resorb. $\underline{7}$ was not clasped since
no suitable undercuts were present. The palate was extended
behind $\underline{3}|$ to reciprocate the bar clasp.

Design B

Plate type major connector was used since the prognosis of some
anterior teeth was dubious, and denture teeth can be more easily
added if adjacent to a metal casting. (In such a case consideration
should be given to an acrylic denture.) $\underline{3}|$ was not clasped since it
was mobile. Reciprocation of $|\underline{4\ 7}$ was obtained by extending the
casting on to the palatal surface.

Instructions to technicians

Only the dental surgeon is in a position to design partial dentures
since only he has access to all the clinical information. The
instructions to the technician must therefore show the design

clearly. Most commercial laboratories provide their own prescription sheets. In most cases these are perfectly adequate as all the relevant information can be included. Written instructions should include:

1. Materials from which denture is to be made.
2. Rests: number and precise position.
3. Clasps: type, number and precise position.
4. Connectors: major and minor.
5. Any other components required such as indirect retainers.
6. Shade and mould of artificial teeth.
7. Any special instructions.

Surveyed casts should be sent with the technical instructions which should include a design sketch. If the precise position of any component is not clear, it should be marked on the stone casts.

Chapter 13

Plastic partial dentures

Many dental surgeons regard the acrylic resin partial denture as a harmful appliance, and use it only because of its low cost. It is often referred to as a 'gum stripper'. Nevertheless over 75% of partial dentures provided in many countries (including the United Kingdom) are constructed of an acrylic base and teeth. However, if care is taken in the design and construction of an acrylic denture, it need not always be a damaging device.

The upper acrylic denture

The prerequisite of a successful mucosa-borne denture is adequate support. The maxilla with its stable hard palate therefore favours the construction of an acceptable mucosa-borne partial denture.

When a mucosa-borne upper partial denture is to be constructed, the most satisfactory design is probably that which follows the principles laid down by Every in 1949. These are:

1. Point contact between natural and artificial teeth.
2. Wide embrasures between adjacent standing and artificial teeth.
3. Free articulation.
4. Uncovered gingivae.
5. Contact with distal surface of last standing tooth.
6. Maximum retention using complete denture principles.

Point contact between natural and artificial teeth (Figure 13.1)

A natural tooth will stand more axial than lateral force. It has been shown that, when periodontal disease is present, lateral force will accelerate periodontal breakdown. By creating a point contact between natural and artificial teeth, lateral forces to standing teeth are minimized and distributed mesiodistally along other teeth in an arch. Note: contact points in the dentate state in the upper arch are situated towards the buccal side of the interproximal area (Figure 13.2).

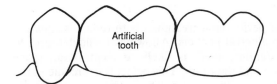

Figure 13.1 Point contacts. Note how interdental gingiva is also cleared

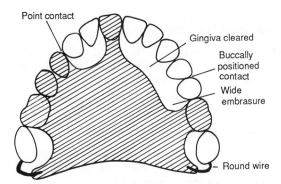

Figure 13.2 Diagram of correct Every denture

Wide embrasures between adjacent natural and artificial teeth

The acrylic base is kept well away from the interproximal area of
natural teeth adjacent to artificial teeth (Figure 13.2). This design
is intended to allow natural stimulation and cleaning of the
gingiva. Wide embrasures also leave fewer stagnation areas. There
is therefore less likelihood of plaque accumulation which
predisposes to periodontal disease or caries.

Free articulation

Again to reduce lateral forces on the denture, and so the standing
teeth, a free articulation is desirable. This has been described as
the type of articulation which permits the mandible to slide from
one position to another, with the upper and lower teeth in contact,
with no tendency for the upper and lower cusps to interlock or
hinder such movement.

Uncovered gingivae

One of the aims of periodontal treatment is to reduce stagnation areas such as deep gingival pockets. Allowing acrylic dentures to abut against the standing teeth is likely to create dead space between the denture and the tooth. This defect is overcome in the Every design by 'clearing' the gingiva. This means that at no point buccally, palatally, or interproximally does acrylic contact the free gingival margin. Palatally the plate should be kept free of the gingiva by at least 3 mm.

Contact with distal surface of last standing tooth

The Every denture is designed to contact the distal surface of the most posterior tooth in the arch on each side. This feature aims to prevent distal drifting of the last standing teeth and so assists the maintenance of arch continuity.

Maximum retention using complete denture principles

Design features which provide optimum retention and stability should be incorporated into the design following the principles adopted for complete dentures (see Chapter 17).

The lower acrylic denture

Indications for the use of an acrylic resin lower partial denture are:

1. Economic factors.
2. Patients with good oral hygiene.
3. Patients with teeth of doubtful prognosis.
4. Teeth on which rests can be placed, i.e. a suitable occlusal surface on a tooth with satisfactory periodontal support.

There are four ways in which a lower acrylic partial denture can damage the mouth:

1. Stripping of gingiva.
2. Damaging lateral forces.
3. An interdental wedging effect.
4. Encouragment of plaque formation.

A lower acrylic partial denture should be constructed so as to eliminate or minimize these damaging features as outlined below (Figure 13.3).

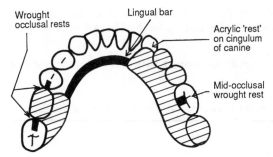

Figure 13.3 Diagram of well constructed acrylic lower partial denture

Elimination of gingival stripping

Effective support by means of rests can be achieved with wrought half round stainless steel wire. The wire must be sufficiently rigid to be effective. For molars 2 mm diameter wire is adequate, whilst for premolars and canines 1.8 mm diameter wire is sufficient.

Support can also be obtained by extending the acrylic above the survey line of a tooth (Figure 13.4) or extending an acrylic lingual plate on to well pronounced cingula of lower incisors. However, these features encourage plaque formation and may subject the teeth to lateral forces.

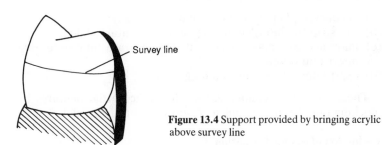

Figure 13.4 Support provided by bringing acrylic above survey line

Avoiding damaging lateral forces

One of the principle design features of the Every acrylic upper denture is that it aims to avoid lateral forces to standing teeth. In a lower plastic partial denture these forces are more difficult to resist. This is because as there is no palate to give rigidity more of the denture must abut against the natural teeth. Wrought rests will usually apply some lateral force to standing teeth during mastication. So will any part of the denture in contact with the lingual or buccal surface of standing teeth. These forces may be reduced by:

1. Having minimal acrylic in contact with the lingual surface of standing teeth.
2. Using as few clasps as possible.
3. Having point contact between natural and artificial teeth.
4. A free articulation.

No interdental wedges

Interdental wedges (Figure 13.5) are often placed on plastic partial dentures to aid retention by wedging into the interdental spaces.

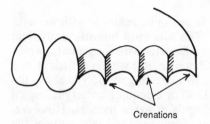

Crenations

Figure 13.5 Crenations (or collets) on a plastic partial denture. These can act as interdental wedges

However they are harmful since they:

(a) encourage plaque formation interproximally;
(b) can strip the interdental gingiva if the denture sinks;
(c) may act as food packers if the denture moves during mastication; and
(d) exert lateral forces on standing teeth.

These should be eliminated on all acrylic partial dentures by blocking out the interdental space on the working model.

Reduction of plaque formation

Several studies have shown that partial dentures encourage plaque formation, particularly on tooth surfaces against which they abut (e.g. Bates and Addy, 1978). Contact of a denture against standing teeth should therefore be minimal. Wrought lingual bars will often avoid the necessity of acrylic abutting the lingual surface of lower teeth. Clasping should be minimal. Oral hygiene instructions should be given *prior* to the construction of all partial dentures, otherwise the denture may not fulfil its function in helping to preserve the remaining teeth.

The acrylic lingual plate

An acrylic lingual plate may be used in some circumstances for, although it encourages plaque formation on the teeth against which it rests, it does have the following advantages:

1. It can provide effective support if the cingula are well developed.
2. If the prognosis of the lower anterior teeth is poor, replacements can easily be added.

The spoon denture

The spoon denture is a satisfactory plastic denture if only one or two anterior teeth need replacement. Its primary use is in children, and in adults as a temporary denture. It should cover a large area of the palate to gain sufficient retention, but the gingiva should not be covered. Its support is gained from the hard palate.

A labial flange may be added to aid retention, but this should engage a precise undercut along a previously surveyed path of insertion.

Chapter 14

Partial dentures for specific problems and relining partial dentures

Lower bilateral free-end saddle

The very nature of this denture creates its own problems, namely:

1. The saddle cannot be fully tooth-supported.
2. The edentulous mucosa must take a high loading.
3. Rotational forces on the abutment teeth, due to saddle sinkage, is hard to avoid.

There are, therefore, three problems to overcome:

1. Obtaining adequate support from the remaining teeth.
2. Preventing rotational forces on the abutment teeth.
3. Obtaining sufficient retention.

Obtaining adequate support

This is achieved by:

1. Utilizing mucosa- and tooth-borne support.
2. Maximum coverage of the edentulous mucosa.
3. Optimum resting, i.e. considering lingual plate or more than two occlusal rests.

Preventing rotational forces on the abutment teeth

Saddle rotation can occur towards the mucosa with masticatory loads (Figure 14.1). or away from the mucosa while chewing sticky foods. Reduction in rotational forces can be achieved in the following ways:

1. By placing the distal rest more anteriorly in the arch and so producing a greater arc of rotation of the saddle (Figure 14.2). This results in a more even loading of the edentulous mucosa.
2. Use of an occlusally approaching clasp with the clasp tips facing towards the saddle (Figure 14.3). Should the saddle lift, the clasps rotate upwards and are opposed by the curvature of the

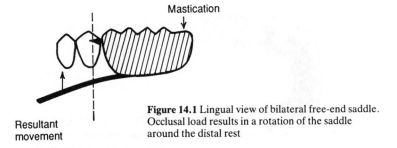

Figure 14.1 Lingual view of bilateral free-end saddle. Occlusal load results in a rotation of the saddle around the distal rest

Resultant movement

Mastication

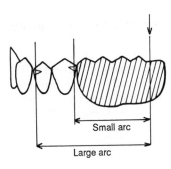

Small arc

Large arc

Figure 14.2 Placing a rest further away from a free-end saddle increases the arc of rotation

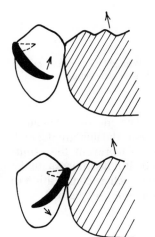

Figure 14.3 The difference between mesially and distally directed clasps in opposing rotation of saddles away from the mucosa

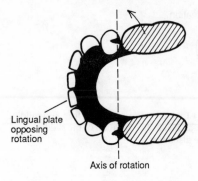

Figure 14.4 An example of indirect retention with a lower free-end saddle. The lingual plate opposes rotational forces

tooth. (Although this system opposes saddle rotation, greater abutment torque may result.)
3. Indirect retention (Figure 14.4).
4. Stress breakers. With a flexible connection between the tooth-supported retaining unit and the saddle there will be a reduction of rotational forces on the abutment teeth (Figure 14.5) (but see Chapter 9, p. 66 for deficiencies of stress breakers).

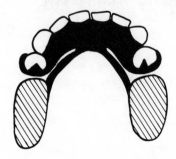

Figure 14.5 Wrought gold lingual bar spot welded to lingual plate acting as stress breaker

5. Using mucocompressive techniques. The mucosa beneath a free-end saddle is subject to displacement; the amount depends on the thickness of the sub-mucosa. To prevent this, some clinicians take impressions of the edentulous mucosa under load with a viscous impression material such as composition or wax (for details of the Applegate technique, see below).

Obtaining sufficient retention

Since only one end of a saddle can be attached to standing teeth, it is often difficult to obtain adequate retention of a free-end saddle.

This problem can be compounded if the crowns of the remaining teeth are conical with insufficient undercuts. Possible solutions include:

1. Clasps. Occlusally approaching clasps usually provide the most effective retention but have poor aesthetic appearance. Gingivally approaching clasps are more widely used. Since the 'angle of removal' for free-end saddles is large (Figure 14.6), it is important that these clasps are placed towards the mesial surface to oppose the distal movement of the saddles.

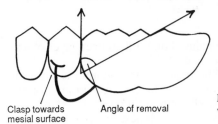

Clasp towards   Angle of removal
mesial surface

Figure 14.6 Large angle of removal with free-end saddles

2. Precision attachments. A wide range of precision attachments specifically designed for free-end saddles is available. However, they have not gained wide acceptance because of the skill and expense involved.
3. Swinglock attachments are not widely used but can be a most useful form of retention (see p. 97).

The Applegate technique

As discussed above, free-end saddles are liable to sink under occlusal pressure because of the displaceability of the mucosa. The Applegate wax displacement technique aims to prevent this by taking an impression of the saddle mucosa under controlled pressure as follows:

1. The metal casting, with temporary self-cured acrylic resin saddles, is tried in. The clearance between saddles and mucosa is 0.25 mm.
2. A viscous impression wax is heated to about 65°C (depending on manufacturers' instructions) and painted onto fitting surface of saddles.
3. The denture is held in place by the metal framework *only*. Finger pressure must *not* be applied to the saddles as this will cause over-displacement of the mucosa.

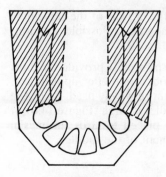

Figure 14.7 Altered cast technique. Shaded area shows portion cut away from master model

4. Further layers of wax are painted on until an even layer of wax with a 'satin finish' is obtained.
5. In the laboratory the saddle region of the denture is cut away from the stone cast (Figure 14.7). The casting is located on the abutment teeth and the saddle impression cast.
6. The saddles are then processed on this new two-part stone cast.

Upper free-end saddle dentures

The problems with this type of prosthesis are similar to a lower free-end saddle denture. The differences are:

1. The palate provides a large area for mucosal support. There is therefore much less tendency for the saddles to sink under load.
2. Retention and stability may be less of a problem because of the large area of denture in contact with the palate. Tongue control is more likely.
3. The upper saddles may fall under the force of gravity.
4. Indirect retention may be difficult to obtain, particularly when the lower incisors occlude on the palatal mucosa. (This prevents anterior extension of the denture.)

Immediate partial dentures

While complete immediate dentures are now becoming less common, immediate partial dentures are being made more often. Instead of extracting all the remaining teeth, only some are removed. The principles of design are the same as for a conventional partial denture. There are some differences in the details and sequence of treatment:

1. At the try-in stage, the replacement artificial teeth cannot be tried in and assessed for shade, occlusion etc.
2. When the teeth to be extracted are removed from the stone master cast, a similar technique to that for complete immediate dentures is followed, i.e. the stone in the area of the extracted teeth should be smooth and rounded, not socketed (Figure 28.2).
3. After extraction of the designated teeth, a rapid phase of healing and localized bone resorption follows. The dentures should therefore be examined frequently and relined when necessary.

More of the population are being rendered edentulous at an advanced age. The immediate partial denture provides a most useful stepping stone to the fully edentulous state. As further teeth are lost they may be added to the (sometimes immediate) partial denture, until eventually the patient has no standing teeth. With this system of the 'creeping denture' they are better able to tolerate the change to complete dentures.

The swinglock attachment

This was introduced in 1963 and its use is taught in more than half the dental schools in the United States. The attachment is preformed in wax and consists of a hinged labial bar which locks into the opposite saddle (Figure 14.8). The labial bar contacts the anterior teeth by means of bar clasps or a shaped labial flange. Only patients with good oral hygiene should be considered for this type of denture.

The advantages of the swinglock system are:

1. Excellent stability and retention are possible.
2. Unsightly gingival recession can be masked with a carefully coloured and contoured flange.

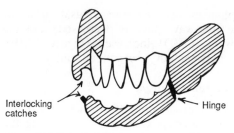

Interlocking catches — Hinge

Figure 14.8 Swinglock denture in open position

Research has shown that caries was rarely a problem in association with this appliance, and tooth mobility was actually found to decrease after a period of use.

The ZA retainer

This attachment was developed in an attempt to overcome the aesthetic problems associated with conventional clasping and the high cost of precision attachments.

The ZA anchor consists of a spring-loaded nylon nipple, contained in a metal casing and grooved for retention (Figure 14.9). It is placed at either end of a bounded saddle so that the

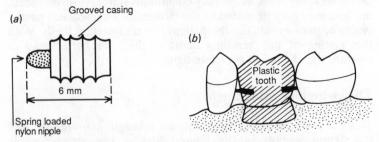

Figure 14.9 ZA anchor: (*a*) close-up of device; (*b*) the device engaging undercuts at both ends of a bounded saddle (survey lines drawn for clarification)

nipple engages the abutment tooth in an undercut region. During insertion and removal the nipple is depressed as the saddle is drawn over the curvature of the abutment teeth. When in place, the nipple should be passive.

Overlays and onlays

These are prosthetic appliances that cover the occlusal surface of the standing teeth. The free-way space is decreased, and the occlusal vertical dimension (OVD) increased (Figure 14.10). There is no difference between an overlay, an onlay and a bite-raising appliance.

Overlays are used in several conditions:

1. Severe attrition, abrasion or erosion. If considerable tooth substance has been lost, overlays can assist in restoring the occlusion, the OVD and improving aesthetics. Furthermore

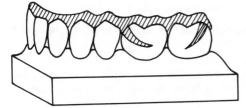

Figure 14.10 Diagram of lower overlay denture

overlays help to prevent further loss of the remaining tooth substance.
2. Temporomandibular joint problems can arise because of a malocclusion. Overlays can help correct severe occlusal abnormalities.
3. Severe malocclusion. The area of interocclusal contact can be greatly increased with overlay dentures.

Sectional dentures

Sectional, or two-part, dentures involve an anterior (or occasionally posterior) flange and teeth which can be separated from the cast metal framework (Figure 14.11). The two parts can be united by a variety of devices. The simplest union is by way of a split post on the cast metal framework which enters a metal tube on the facade. Since the two parts of the denture have two different paths of insertion, great retention is possible. Furthermore unsightly gingiva, teeth and bony 'undercuts' can be covered since a horizontal path of insertion of the flange may be used.

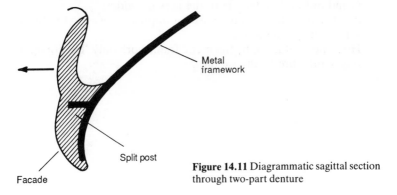

Metal framework

Split post

Facade

Figure 14.11 Diagrammatic sagittal section through two-part denture

The advantages of sectional dentures are therefore:

1. Aesthetics can be better since no clasps need to be used anteriorly.
2. Retention is superior.
3. Bony undercuts which cannot be filled with a conventional denture can be filled with a flange having a horizontal path of insertion.

Relining partial dentures

The relining of partial dentures is often a more difficult procedure than the relining of complete dentures. This is because the reline impression material may flow into undercuts of the standing teeth, and when replaced with acrylic resin lining the denture becomes difficult or impossible to fit. Unfortunately many practitioners insert partial dentures relined by this method and adjust by eye until the denture can be inserted. This results in a partial denture that does not fit accurately around the standing teeth.

For mucosa-supported acrylic dentures, often the most efficient way to reline them is to take an impression of the partially dentate mouth and reline the denture on properly blocked-out stone casts. This method only works if the denture can be correctly positioned on the blocked-out cast – not always the case. Because of this many clinicians advocate remaking rather than relining mucosa-borne dentures.

Cast metal dentures are usually easier to reline since the acrylic saddle does not abut against an undercut region of the standing teeth. The reline procedure is as follows:

1. Check the extension of the saddles; correct if necessary.
2. Grind out any undercuts in the acrylic saddle.
3. Apply zinc oxide/eugenol paste or impression wax to the fitting surface of the denture.
4. Hold the denture in by the metal framework only. Do not apply finger pressure to the saddles.

Chapter 15

Resin retained bridges

General description

Resin retained bridges (also called adhesive bridges) require very little tooth preparation. The artificial tooth (pontic) is held in place by retainers (or wings) which are cemented to the adjacent teeth with a composite resin. The enamel of the retaining teeth is acid-etched to increase the adhesion (Figure 15.1).

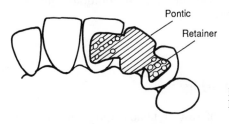

Pontic

Retainer

Figure 15.1 Palatal view of upper Rochette bridge

The uses of resin retained bridges are:

1. To replace missing teeth.
2. Splinting, for periodontal or orthodontic purposes.

Advantages of resin retained bridges

The advantages are:

1. No or very little tooth preparation needed.
2. No danger of involving the dental pulp – especially useful in young teeth or lower incisors.
3. No anaesthesia required.
4. No metal margins likely to cause gingival irritation.
5. Minimal or no mucosal coverage – in contrast to partial dentures.
6. Essentially a reversible procedure.
7. Cheaper than conventional bridges.

Disadvantages of resin retained bridges

The disadvantages are:

1. Must have sound adjacent enamel on which retainers can be cemented.
2. Failure of an abutment tooth usually necessitates completely remaking bridge.
3. The bridges often cannot withstand high masticatory stresses and are therefore unsuitable for the replacement of teeth subjected to heavy stresses.

Indications for a resin retained bridge

The indications are:

1. Small edentulous span.
2. Sound abutment teeth without large restorations and with enamel suitable for bonding.
3. Good oral hygiene.
4. Favourable occlusion.

Types of resin retained bridge

There are two main types of resin retained bridge in use – the Rochette and the Maryland.

The Rochette bridge

The Rochette technique was first described in the early 1970s as a periodontal splint. Other clinicians soon modified the splint to form a bridge. The adhesion of the bridge is increased by 6–10 perforations in each retainer unit. These are conical with the apex toward the enamel so as to provide mechanical retention (Figure 15.2).

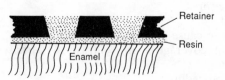

Figure 15.2 Diagrammatic cross-section of Rochette bridge retainer

Advantages of Rochette bridge

1. Easy to remove and if necessary recement.
2. Contamination of metal fitting surface during cementation less likely to affect retention.

A Rochette bridge is removed by drilling the resin from the retaining holes, and then tapping the bridge with an impact type crown remover.

The Maryland bridge

The composite gains its retention from electrolytic etching of the retainer's fitting surface, a system described as micromechanical retention. There are no holes in the retaining units (Figure 15.3).

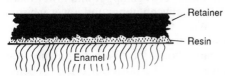

Figure 15.3 Diagrammatic cross-section of Maryland bridge retainer

Some laboratories now obtain a retentive roughness of the fitting surface of Maryland bridges by covering the fitting surface with minute beads or meshes at the wax-up stage, or alternatively metal substances may be added to the surface after casting and then sintering in a furnace.

Advantages of Maryland bridge

1. Greater retention than Rochette bridge.
2. Smooth lingual or palatal surface of retainer.
3. Stronger. (Rochette bridges are weakened by their retaining holes.)

Technique for the construction of resin retained bridges

There are six clinical stages in the construction of a resin retained bridge:

1. Patient selection.
2. Design.
3. Tooth preparation.
4. Impressions.
5. Try-in.
6. Cementation.

Patient selection

A number of factors must be considered in assessing the suitability of a patient for an adhesive bridge:

1. The space to be filled: generally only one or two unit spaces are available.
2. The retaining teeth: must be healthy and have sufficient enamel for bonding.
3. Prognosis of other teeth in the arch: if nearby teeth are likely to be lost, a partial denture may be a more suitable long-term replacement.
4. Occlusion: when replacing anterior teeth the incisal relationship should be studied. Points to note include the space available for the retaining units between upper and lower teeth in occlusion, and the relation between upper and lower incisors in eccentric movements. Wear facets on incisors and canines often indicate a powerful protrusive movement of the lower incisors; in these cases care should be taken to balance the bridge for protrusive movements. If a posterior bridge is being considered, the occlusion must be studied to ensure the bridge will withstand the masticatory forces.
5. The oral hygiene must be satisfactory. Most resin retained bridges create a space between the pontic and retainer which requires a special cleaning technique.

Design of the bridge

The points to be considered when designing a resin retained bridge are:

1. The path of insertion. In conventional bridge preparation great emphasis is placed on parallelism of the preparations, and the surface area of the prepared tooth in contact with the retaining unit. These features are also important with resin retained bridges. Surveyed study models will indicate the need or desirability of grinding enamel to increase the area in contact with the retaining unit (Figure 15.4).

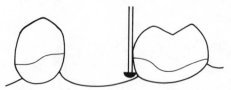

Figure 15.4 Diagram of surveyed teeth. Undercut gauge indicates amount of enamel that needs to be ground to remove interproximal undercut

2. The size and shape of the retaining wings. On anterior teeth the
    retaining wings should be about 2 mm short of the incisal edge
    to avoid loss of the natural translucency. The base of the
    retainer should clear the gingival margin by about 0.5 mm
    (Figure 15.5). In posterior teeth the area of retainer is often
    influenced by the palatal bulge (Figure 15.6). If the survey line
    is too high it may be lowered by grinding.

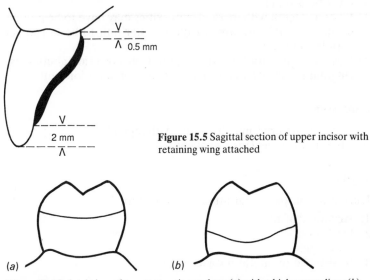

Figure 15.5 Sagittal section of upper incisor with retaining wing attached

Figure 15.6 Palatal view of two contrasting molars: (*a*) with a high survey line; (*b*) with a low survey line. Enamel on (*a*) may need to be ground to lower survey line

Particularly in posterior teeth, a wrap-around retainer, i.e
one that covers the mesial, lingual, and distal surface of a
retaining tooth, will increase resistance to lateral displacement
(Figure 15.7).

Retainers need to be 0.5 mm thick except in areas of high
stress, e.g. where the retainer joins the pontic. Here 1 mm
thickness is required.

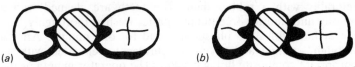

Figure 15.7 Occlusal view of posterior bridges. Retainers in (*a*) cover minimum of
lingual enamel. Retainers in (*b*) have wrap-around extension and provide greater
resistance to lateral displacement

Tooth preparation

Removal of some surface enamel may be required for a number of reasons:

1. With upper anterior bridges there must be sufficient clearance between the upper and lower incisors. If there is insufficient room either the upper palatal surface or the lower incisal edges must be ground.
2. Posterior teeth with marked convexities may have to be ground to allow a sufficient area of the retainer unit to be in contact with the enamel.
3. Rest seat preparations are required on posterior abutments; cingulum rests are occasionally needed on anterior teeth.

Impressions

Any elastic material may be used. Although elastomers are most suitable, many clinicians use alginate.

Try-in

During try-in, particular attention is paid to:

1. Accuracy of fit.
2. Occlusion.
3. Aesthetics.
4. Resistance to lateral displacement.

After the try-in, the fitting surface of the retaining units must be meticulously cleaned if they have been contaminated with saliva. A solvent such as chloroform is effective. This is particularly critical with the Maryland bridge which relies on micromechanical retention. Some clinicians have the fitting surface of the Maryland bridge re-etched after the try-in. A further appointment is then required to cement the bridge.

Cementation

For cementation, the retaining teeth must be well isolated, preferably with a rubber dam. The teeth are cleaned with a non-oily and fluoride-free pumice paste, washed thoroughly, and then etched with 37% phosphoric acid for one minute. After a thorough washing and drying the bridge is cemented with an appropriate composite luting cement. The operator maintains the position of the bridge while he, or an assistant, removes excess cement.

During trimming and polishing, after the cement has set, care should be taken to avoid overheating the metal framework, which will damage the composite cement.

Since the precise seating of anterior bridges can be difficult, some laboratories provide incisive hooks for correct positioning. After cementing, these hooks are removed with fine diamond burs and the edges polished.

Materials used in the construction of resin bonded bridges

The metal framework of a resin retained bridge may be constructed of gold alloy or a semi-precious material. With the Maryland technique, it is important that the metal used has the correct etching characteristics. The pontic is usually made of bonding porcelain, but may be made of acrylic.

Complete dentures

Chapter 16

Impressions

An impression aims to record the oral tissues in such a way as to produce maximum retention and stability in the completed denture.

Retention is defined as the resistance of a denture to displacement in an occlusal direction.

Stability is defined as the resistance of a denture to displacement by functional stress. By implication stability primarily resists horizontal forces (Figure 16.1).

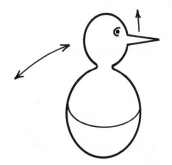

Figure 16.1 Weighted plastic toy illustrating difference between retention and stability. Resistance to vertical displacement (retention) is small, but after being pushed laterally the bird returns to vertical (good stability)

The neutral zone: stability is aided by muscle balance where the lips, cheeks and tongue do not act to displace the denture during function. This muscle balance is achieved when the denture is placed within the neutral zone (also called the zone of minimum conflict or denture space). When natural teeth erupt, they are guided into the neutral zone by the adjacent muscles, i.e. the tongue on one side and the cheeks and lips on the other. Artificial teeth should be placed within this zone so that they are not unduly acted on by any muscle group.

The shape of the polished surface is an important factor in denture stability. If correctly shaped the adjacent muscles will stabilize and not displace the denture. In the upper denture the buccal surfaces should incline downwards and outwards. This enables the buccinator to push the upper denture towards the

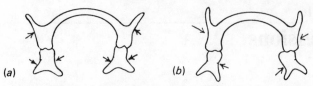

Figure 16.2 Section through complete dentures: (*a*) correctly shaped polished surfaces with stabilizing muscle forces (arrowed); (*b*) incorrectly shaped polished surfaces. Muscle forces (arrowed) act to dislodge dentures

supporting tissues (Figure 16.2). If the upper buccal surface sloped in the opposite direction, the buccinator would probably displace the upper denture. Similarly with the lower denture, the lingual surface should face upwards and inwards. This enables the tongue to stabilize the denture. Furthermore the buccal surfaces should face upwards and outwards to transmit the stabilizing forces of the cheek muscles.

Resistance to displacement: in practice it is often hard to differentiate between stability and retention, a fact that has led to much confused thinking. The authors believe it is better to combine the two terms into 'resistance to displacement'. Factors which are involved in the resistance to displacement of complete dentures may be divided into:

1. Physical factors, e.g. cohesion (the forces of attraction between like molecules); adhesion (the forces of attraction between unlike molecules); surface tension of saliva; the viscosity of saliva; and gravity.
2. Mechanical factors, which involve primarily the engagement of soft tissue undercuts.
3. Physiological factors relating to the action of the muscles. The muscles of the lips, cheeks and tongue should not act to displace dentures during function and, indeed, correct shaping of polished surfaces of a denture may aid resistance to displacement. Futhermore, occlusal balance should be such that during mastication one denture should move over the other without tending to displace either denture.

In practice, maximum resistance to displacement of a complete denture is obtained if the following six features are incorporated:

1. Optimum extension of the denture base.
2. As close an adaptation of the denture base to the oral mucosa as possible.
3. An effective peripheral seal.

4. Polished surfaces shaped to aid muscle control.
5. Teeth placed within the neutral zone.
6. A balanced articulation.

Primary impressions

Primary impressions may be taken in any impression material, provided that it records the denture-bearing area sufficiently well to enable construction of a suitable special tray. The primary impression should reproduce:

1. The sulcus depth.
2. The sulcus width along the entire periphery.
3. Certain anatomical landmarks which indicate the correct extension of the special tray, e.g. foveae palatinae and retromolar pads.

Any impression materal may be used for primary impressions, but in dental schools composition is the most popular because it can easily be adapted should the first attempt at impressions be unsuccessful. Note: when using impression compound, it should be heated in a water bath at 60–65°C and kneaded well. Water incorporated within the material acts as a plasticizer.

Alginate, plaster or elastomers should be considered if:

1. Undercuts are present.
2. There is a flabby ridge.

Primary impressions are taken in stock trays. When trying in a stock tray prior to impression taking, the following points should be noted:

1. The flanges do not impinge on any fraena.
2. There is no space between tray and mucosa.
3. The upper tray extends round the maxillary tuberosity.
4. The lower tray extends over the retromolar pad.

The importance of sulcus width

Certain impression techniques require a registration of the sulcus width so as to provide maximum retention and stability.

A good peripheral seal can be more easily obtained if the entire sulcal width is filled (Figure 16.3). This is because the tissues of the sulcus, which form a seal with the periphery of the denture, contact a far larger area of the denture if the sulcus is completely filled.

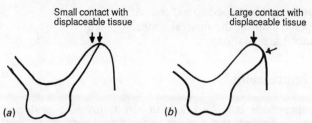

Figure 16.3 To illustrate how a denture periphery which fills the sulcus creates better retention: (*a*) diagrammatic cross-section through upper denture with small area of peripheral contact; (*b*) fully filled sulcus and large area of peripheral contact with displaceable tissue.

Greater stability is also obtained when the sulcus is fully filled. Firstly, this is because it is easier to form the polished surfaces into the most efficient shape to aid stability (Figure 16.4) and, secondly, by filling the mandibular buccal sulcus the lower denture is more able to resist occlusal tipping forces (Figure 16.5).

Sulcus width is most easily recorded with a primary composition impression and by constructing a special tray of the correct thickness. Alternatively the sulcus width can be recorded by adding green stick composition, carding wax, etc. to the periphery of the special tray.

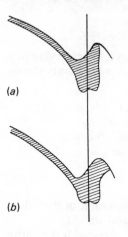

Figure 16.4 If true breadth of buccal sulcus is not reproduced with teeth placed in correct position, polished surface may not have optimal shape (compare *a* and *b*)

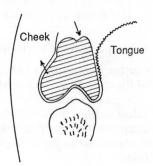

Figure 16.5 Fully filled mandibular sulcus resists occlusal tipping forces

Special impression trays

Special impression trays may be constructed in shellac or plastic.
No separation between cast and special tray is required for:

1. Zinc oxide pastes, with or without eugenol.
2. Impression wax.

Separations commonly used for the following materials are:

1. Plaster – 2 mm.
2. Alginate with tray perforations – 3 mm.
3. Elastomeric materials – 1.5 mm.

Effect of muscles on impression form

Certain muscles will affect the form and depth of the sulcus,
should they be active during impression taking:

1. Swallowing: the tongue is raised by the mylohyoid during
   swallowing; this makes the mandibular distolingual sulcus
   shallower.
2. Protrusion of the tongue also reduces the depth of the lingual
   sulcus because of contraction of the myohyoid and genioglossus
   muscles.
3. The orbicularis oris can easily displace an excessively thick
   labial flange. However these movements do not affect the
   depth of the labial sulcus.
4. Buccinator contraction does not affect sulcus depth but it
   reduces width.

Impression techniques

There is a wide variety of techniques described for taking
secondary impressions. The fact that no one technique is
universally performed suggests that none is consistently superior.

The closed mouth technique

With this method, impressions are taken within the trial denture or
within occlusal rims on a rigid base. Upper and lower impressions
are taken together. Impressions are taken with the dentures or
rims in retruded contact position (RCP).

It is claimed that this technique minimizes slight occlusal errors caused by differential displacement of the mucosa because, while the dentures are in occlusion, any slight discrepancies in the evenness of contact between denture base and mucosa is taken up by the impression material. For a full description of this technique see Farrell (1976).

Half-open mouth technique

Some clinicians believe that this is the most relevant record, since it is the most frequent position of the mouth during speech and in opening while eating. Many practitioners of this method ask the patient to protrude the tongue slightly while the lower impression is being taken.

Fully open mouth impressions

These record the mouth when the dentures are potentially most unretentive.

Functional impressions

These are recorded while the patient moves the musculature so as to imitate functional movements such as pursing the lips, opening and closing the mouth, and swallowing. Impressions may also be taken over many days with a functional impression material used inside a set of old dentures. Some operators pull gently on the lips and cheeks during impression taking to mimic a natural muscular movement.

Faults to avoid with impressions

The most common faults which should be avoided are:

1. Under-extension, seen as feather-edging of periphery (Figure 16.6).
2. Tissue displacement: tray shows through impression.
3. Over-extension: periphery of tray shows through impression.
4. Air and saliva bubbles: most detrimental at the periphery.
5. Trapping of tongue or cheek.
6. Excessive mucus: seen mainly on posterior palatal portion of upper impression.
7. Separation of material from tray, especially from heel of lower tray.

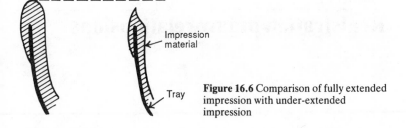

Figure 16.6 Comparison of fully extended impression with under-extended impression

Special techniques

Special impression techniques are required for flabby ridges and certain oral defects such as cleft palates.

The flabby ridge

Particular care must be taken not to displace a flabby ridge while taking impressions for subsequent dentures may be unstable due to pressure from the stressed ridge.

Many techniques have been described for impressions of flabby ridges. In essence, all require a very fluid material so that the ridge is not displaced. One commonly used technique uses a special tray with a window through which the ridge hangs. An impression of the firm tissues is first taken in the special tray with zinc oxide and eugenol paste. Plaster is then painted on to the flabby ridge hanging through the tray. When set the two-part impression is removed as one, a stock tray enclosing both parts.

Cleft palates, fistulae and surgical spaces

These create special problems as they may become filled with impression material which is difficult or impossible to remove. If an impression of the defect cavity is not required, it must be temporarily filled to prevent impression material lodging in it. Dental gauze lubricated with petroleum jelly is usually sufficient.

Chapter 17

Registration of jaw relationships

Jaw relationships are discussed in Chapter 3. With complete dentures most prosthetists consider it best to record the retruded contact position (RCP), as opposed to muscle position, because it is constant and easily reproducible. Since many patients will reflexly occlude into the muscle position which is 0–1.2 mm anterior to RCP, it is important to achieve a balance between these two positions – a situation sometimes called 'long centric'.

The clinical measurement of RCP is most important. If it is not correct complete dentures, satisfactory in all other respects, may be unwearable. The registration of RCP is divided into:

1. The measurement of occlusal vertical dimension (OVD).
2. The recording of horizontal jaw relationship.

Clinical methods of measuring occlusal vertical dimension (OVD)

Most clinical methods of measuring OVD are based on measuring the rest vertical dimension (RVD) and reducing this by 2–4 mm to provide sufficient free-way space.

Instruments for measuring OVD include:

1. Willis bite gauge.
2. Callipers.
3. Screw jack.

Willis bite gauge

The Willis bite gauge (or more correctly the Willis gauge) measures the distance between the base of the nose and the underside of the chin (Figure 17.1). Since both these features are displaceable, considerable skill is needed to obtain consistent results. McMillan and Imber (1968) showed that few operators were able to repeat results to within + or − 1 mm.

Other more complex gauges have been developed, e.g. the dakometer and the Chick gauge. However these have not been generally accepted.

Callipers

Callipers measure the distance between two markings, one on the point of the chin and the other on the tip of the nose (Figure 17.2). This method probably gives more consistent results than the Willis gauge.

Both the Willis gauge and callipers can only be as accurate as the soft tissues permit (Figure 17.3).

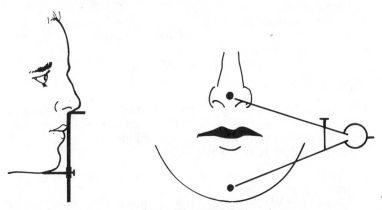

Figure 17.1 Willis gauge in use   **Figure 17.2** Callipers in use

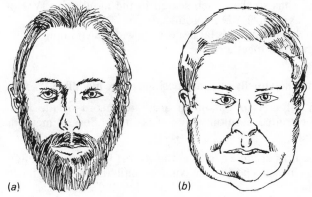

(a)   (b)

Figure 17.3 In patient (a) a calliper reading is difficult. In patient (b) a Willis gauge reading is difficult

Screw jack

This consists of an adjustable screw fitted onto one base-plate and bearing onto the opposing base plate. Patients are thus able to adjust their own vertical dimension until they feel comfortable. With cooperative patients a consistent and acceptable OVD is produced.

Methods of determining jaw relationships

The following methods may be used to determine RCP:

1. Occlusal rims.
2. Copying existing dentures.
3. Using existing occlusion (immediate dentures).
4. Gothic arch tracing device.

Occlusal rims

The successful recording of RCP depends on first obtaining occlusal vertical dimension (OVD) and then recording the most retruded unstrained position of the mandible.

The procedure is as follows:

1. The patient should be seated in an upright position and in a relaxed frame of mind.
2. Measure RVD with one rim in place (the lower rim is sometimes used as there is evidence that it produces a gravity effect on mandibular position).
3. Trim the rims so that when seated in the mouth an OVD of 2–4 mm less than RVD is produced.
4. Retrude the mandible as far as possible without straining it, and locate the rims together.

Obtaining the maximally retruded position of the mandible

It is often difficult to obtain an accurate record of the most unstrained retruded position with occlusal rims. Several methods may be used:

1. Once the rims occlude evenly at the correct OVD, the patient is asked to close in a position of comfort until 'the teeth just touch each other'.
2. When the patient tends to protrude the jaw, a small piece of wax is placed on the posterior border of the upper base. The

patient is asked to touch this with the tip of the tongue, and keep it there while biting gently together.

3. Gentle but firm pressure may be applied to the chin or angles of the mandible. This is effective only if the patient is relaxed and the mandible can be moved freely by the operator. (Relaxation can usually be obtained by asking the patient to 'get the jaw loose and floppy'.)

4. Finally in some cases it has been found that asking the patient to 'push out the upper teeth' may be useful.

Location of rims

After RCP has been ascertained, the rims will need to be located or fixed in this position. This can be achieved by:

1. Cutting notches in the upper and lower rims and recording the relationship with plaster or wax.

2. Applying zinc oxide/eugenol impression paste onto the occlusal surfaces and allowing it to set with the rims in RCP.

3. Stapling the rims together with U-shaped wires or copper rings, heated sufficiently to soften the wax rim.

4. Warming the occlusal surface of both rims, so that they fuse together. (Caution: OVD may be affected.)

Copying existing dentures (see also p. 188)

If the patient is wearing dentures with satisfactory aesthetics, vertical dimension and jaw relationships, a copy denture technique may be used. Strictly speaking muscular position is more likely to be reproduced in such cases.

Using existing occlusion

If sufficient teeth are in occlusion prior to extraction, the jaw relationship may be copied (in this case one is copying PMI). Even if fewer teeth are present there may be occlusal stops – useful for obtaining OVD.

Gothic arch tracing devices

This procedure is based on the principle that the maximum retruded position can be obtained by tracing mandibular movements.

The apparatus consists essentially of an intra- or extra-oral stylus attached to the maxillary rim and a plate attached to the

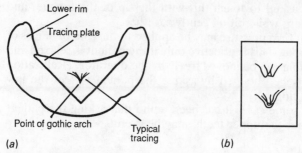

Figure 17.4 (*a*) Gothic arch tracing plate fixed to lower rim. (*b*) Examples of tracing of no clinical value as a gothic point has not been obtained

mandibular rim (Figure 17.4). When the patient moves the lower jaw from side to side a gothic arch is traced on the plate. This arch only forms a sharp apex when the jaw moves through the maximally retruded position.

When a satisfactory tracing has been obtained, a perspex disc with a small hole is attached to the tracing plate. The hole is centred over the apex of the gothic arch. The patient is then instructed to occlude until the stylus locates in the perspex hole, i.e. at RCP. The upper and lower rims are secured with a generous quantity of plaster.

Common causes of error

Common causes of error in recording RCP are:

1. Non-retentive or unstable base plates.
2. Unequal pressure when rims occlude. Rims must meet evenly. Recording material must be evenly softened.
3. Mandible not fully retruded.
4. Premature contact of bases between retromolar pad and tuberosity.

The use of occlusal pivots

Sometimes complete denture wearers develop a habit posture. This is an occlusal relationship that is considerably different from RCP. It occurs especially when the occlusal surface is severely worn, allowing the lower jaw to posture anteriorly. In these patients the recording of RCP can be very difficult. Furthermore, even if RCP can be recorded, new dentures may be uncomfortable as the patient tends to adopt into the habit posture.

This is dealt with by using temporary occlusal pivots before constructing new dentures. Self-curing acrylic resin is added to the occlusal surface in the region of the lower second premolar and first molar; the upper denture then occludes with the resin pivots. After wearing the modified denture for two weeks, the occlusion will gradually return to near RCP.

Summary of clinical procedure

The clinical procedure for registering RCP with occlusal rims is as follows:

1. Trim upper occlusal rim:
   (a) Obtain correct lip support (see Chapter 19).
   (b) Allow 0–2 mm of rim to show below upper lip. (In the elderly less of the upper teeth show, but more of the lower are visible.)
   (c) Ensure that upper rim is parallel with interpupillary line (Figure 17.5).

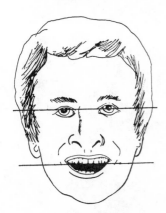

Figure 17.5 Occlusal plane parallel with interpupillary line

   (d) Trim entire rim so that the occlusal plane lies midway between edentulous ridges. (Ala-tragal line, also called Camper's plane, is usually parallel with the occlusal plane in the natural dentition. Many clinicians use this as a guide.)
   (e) Mark midline. Some clinicians also mark lip line and position of canines.

2. Trim lower occlusal rim:
   (a) Obtain correct lip support.
   (b) Trim so that opposing occlusal surfaces meet evenly and that there is a free-way space of 2–4 mm.
3. Locate rims in RCP.

Chapter 18

Articulators

An articulator is a mechanical device that represents the temporomandibular joint and jaws, to which the upper and lower casts may be attached.

It is often stated that the patient is the best articulator; however, mechanical alternatives are most useful and are often a less troublesome substitute. It must be remembered, however, that even the most sophisticated articulator is limited in its ability to reproduce the jaw movements.

Uses

The uses of articulators are:

1. Diagnosis and treatment planning.
2. To facilitate technical procedures for complete and removable partial dentures, and for advanced restorative work.

Definitions

The following definitions are used in the discussion of articulators.

Condylar guide

The device on an articulator which produces movement similar to the paths of the condyles in the temporomandibular joint. The condylar guidance angle or inclination is the angle of this guide to the horizontal plane.

Incisal guidance

This is the influence which the upper and lower anterior teeth have over mandibular movements. The incisal guidance angle is that

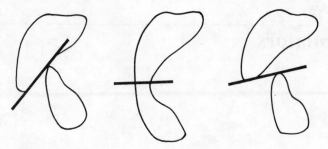

Figure 18.1 Variation in incisor relationship affecting incisal guidance

angle formed with the horizontal plane by drawing a line in the sagittal plane between the incisal edges of upper and lower incisors when the teeth are in RCP (Figure 18.1).

Incisal guidance is usually set at 10° and seldom more than 20° for complete dentures. The incisal guidance angle *increases* as the overbite increases but *decreases* as the overjet increases. Thus if a deep overbite is required for aesthetic reasons, the overjet must be increased to keep the incisal guidance within reasonable limits.

Bennett angle (or horizontal condylar angle)

This is the angle created by the path of the advancing condyle in the sagittal plane during lateral movements.

Bennett shift

This is the bodily lateral movement of the mandible 1–2 mm towards the working side. It is caused by the action of the lateral pterygoid on the condyle of the balancing side.

Arcon construction

Most articulators have the condylar ball attached to the upper arm (e.g. Dentatus ARL, Hanau H2). Arcon articulators have the condylar ball attached to the lower member. It has been claimed that this principle, which copies the arrangement of the temporomandibular joint, has advantages over the more common type. However, mathematical analysis has disproved this.

Classification

It is very difficult to classify articulators as there is often a degree of overlap between the groups. However, accepting this draw-back, the following simple classification is suggested:

1. Simple hinge.
2. Mean value.
3. Semi-adjustable.
4. Fully adjustable.

Simple hinge

Most popular articulator in the UK, not only for prosthetic work but also for more advanced restorative procedures. It does not produce functional movements. Used if occlusal contacts are to be perfect in PMI only.

Mean value

These instruments allow lateral and protrusive movements based on average determinations, i.e. condylar guidance angle and incisive guidance are fixed, the values usually being 30° and 10° respectively. The casts are usually mounted arbitrarily on the instrument (e.g. Simplex).

Semi-adjustable

Such devices will accept facebow transfer and interocclusal records can be used to record the condylar angle (e.g. Dentatus ARL, Hanau H2) (Figure 18.2).

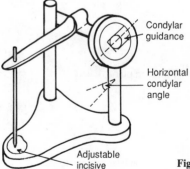

Figure 18.2 Typical features found on semi-adjustable articulator

Fully adjustable

These are capable of reproducing jaw movements with great accuracy. They are usually programmed using dynamic functional recordings. (All determinants taken for the semi-adjustable are static border movement records which may well be outside the normal functional range of jaw movements.) These instruments are normally of the arcon type.

Facebow

The facebow is a calliper-like device used to record the relationship of the maxilla to the terminal hinge axis of the condyles (commonly called the condylar axis) (Figures 18.3 and 18.4).

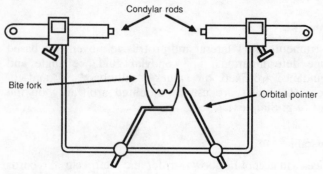

Condylar rods

Bite fork

Orbital pointer

Figure 18.3 The facebow

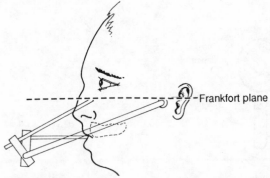

Frankfort plane

Figure 18.4 Use of facebow to relate maxilla to the condylar axis and to the Frankfort plane

The typical facebow has three functions:

1. To relate the maxilla to the terminal hinge axis of the condyles.
2. To relate the occlusal plane to the Frankfort plane, i.e. it relates the occlusal plane to the horizontal plane.
3. To facilitate mounting the casts onto an articulator.

There are two main types of facebow – the arbitrary axis and the kinematic.

Arbitrary axis facebow

This type is considered adequate for prosthetic work. It basically consists of a U-shaped frame with condylar pins located at the ends of the frame. To this a fork is attached which locates to the upper jaw. Often an orbital pointer relates the bow to the Frankfort plane. There are two subdivisions:

1. Facial type bow. The condyles are located arbitrarily by marking a point 13 mm in front of the most distal part of the tragus along a line to the outer canthus of the eye (Figure 18.5).

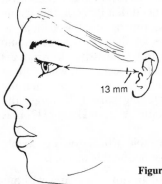

13 mm

Figure 18.5 Arbitrary hinge axis

2. The ear piece bow. This has the condylar pins located in the external auditory meatus. On being transferred to the articulator, locators compensate for the fact that the meatus is posterior to the retruded condylar head.

Kinematic bow

If great accuracy is necessary, for example with complex crown and bridge work, a kinematic record is preferable. This has a fork which is fixed to the lower teeth. This fork is attached to a frame with adjustable points which can be arbitrarily positioned over the condyles. The patient is asked to make small opening and closing movements and the pointers are adjusted until no translation occurs, i.e. there is purely rotational movement. This hinge axis is marked with a skin marking pencil and the bow is then used in a regular manner, being fastened into place over these recorded points.

Choice of articulator for prosthetic work

Dentures made in general practice in many countries are constructed on simple hinge articulators to the satisfaction of most patients.

Once food is introduced it is impossible to maintain balancing contacts until the bolus of food is broken down to small pieces, when it would appear that the position a patient tends to find at the end of a chewing cycle is RCP. Some workers consider that as long as the teeth are set in this retruded contact position (by means of a simple hinge articulator), the dentures can be satisfactory and any movement not permitted by the occlusion the patient will avoid. However, it can be strongly argued that it is not reasonable to construct such limiting dentures, relying on the patient to compensate for inherent deficiencies in their prosthesis. Some patients need to perform lateral and protrusive movements without interfence and it seems that a free occlusion, where there are no interfering contacts, is a sensible aim. It is generally accepted that for denture work, including partial dentures, the semi-adjustable articulator, e.g. Dentatus ARL or Hanau H2, is as complicated as is necessary.

The high accuracy of the fully adjustable articulator is probably not relevant to prosthetic work. Reasons for this include:

1. The oral mucosa can be displaced by up to 0.5 mm without undue force. If this displacement were to occur in both jaws, errors up to 1 mm might occur.
2. Few technicians can position casts consistently on an articulator. In one study (Watt, 1968) 30 identical casts were mounted on the same articulator using a special rigid jig. Even with this fixed mounting, errors greater than 1 mm were found in the vertical plane.
3. Clinical studies have been conducted comparing complete dentures made on a simple adjustable articulator with those made on a fully adjustable instrument. No superiority could be demonstrated for those dentures made on the more complex articulator.

Monson's sphero-ellipsoidal theory

Monson observed that the occlusal surfaces of the posterior teeth lay on an upward curve, the radius of which was 4 inches (Figure 18.6). Von Spee had earlier described the anterior-posterior curve of the occlusal table. Monson's spheroidal plate was designed so that the artificial teeth would conform to these curves. The limitations of this technique are that it does not allow for any vertical incisal overlap and *only* cuspless teeth can be used if the articulation is to be balanced. Some dental laboratories still use curved plates to assist them in setting up teeth.

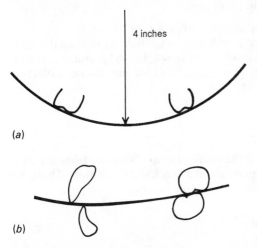

(a)

(b)

Figure 18.6 (*a*) Curve of Monson. (*b*) Effect of setting up to Monson's spheroidal plates: incisors have no vertical overlap

Chapter 19

Setting up the teeth

The aim of setting up teeth

The aims of setting up teeth are:

1. To create a natural pleasing appearance.
2. To make the dentures as stable as possible by placing the teeth in the neutral zone, and correctly shaping the polished surfaces.
3. To establish a balanced articulation for masticatory efficiency and denture stability.

Facial form

Before recording RCP the occlusal rims should be trimmed so as to support the facial musculature in a natural position. There are several guides which may be useful for this:

1. Naso-labial angle.
2. Lip-cheek junction.
3. Anterior lip plane.

Naso-labial angle

In most patients the sagittal naso-labial angle is 90° (Figure 19.1). However, if the patient has a snub or hooked nose the angle may have to be modified. Also if the patient's natural upper incisors are retroclined, a more obtuse angle will usually appear natural.

It should also be noted that the naso-labial angle is affected by labial contouring of the *whole* upper rim and the OVD which, as it is increased, causes the angle to become more obtuse.

The lip-cheek junction

The upper lip should merge imperceptibly with the cheek. If a fold develops between the two, there may be insufficient support of the entire upper lip (Figure 19.2).

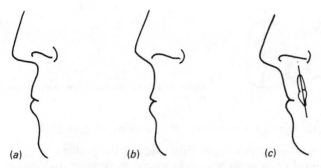

Figure 19.1 Variations in naso-labial angle: (*a*) conventional 90° angle; (*b*) snub nose and an obtuse angle; (*c*) retroclined upper incisors and an obtuse angle

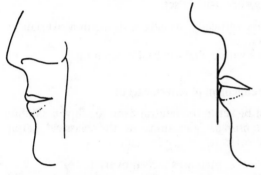

Figure 19.2 Unwanted fold between upper lip and cheek

Figure 19.3 With most patients the upper and lower lip are in the same plane

Anterior lip plane

In most cases the lower lip should protrude almost as much as the upper lip. If not, this is usually due to inadequate lower lip support or to insufficient vertical dimension (Figure 19.3). In certain ethnic groups, e.g. negroes, the lips may remain competent and well supported even in the absence of anterior teeth.

Setting up anterior teeth

When setting up anterior teeth, the labial form should be maintained since the rims should have already been moulded to provide a pleasing facial form. Usually the upper anteriors are set up before the lower anteriors.

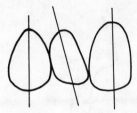

Figure 19.4 Angulations of upper incisors and canines

The *upper anterior* are usually set as follows (Figure 19.4):

1. The central incisors vertical either side of the midline.
2. The lateral incisors with a slight mesial inclination and about 1 mm shorter than the centrals.
3. The canines vertical, often with necks slightly labially inclined.

The *lower anteriors* are usually set:

1. The lower incisors vertically, usually with a 3 mm overlap by the upper incisors.
2. The lower canines with a slight mesial inclination.

Variations in the arrangement of anterior teeth

Artificial teeth must be set in the neutral zone to allow maximum stability for the dentures. Variations in the classical set-up described above are often necessary to achieve this:

1. Angle Class II, div. 1: increases incisal overjet.
2. Angle Class II, div. 2: increased vertical overlap with retro-inclination of the upper incisors. However if any protrusive balance is required, the vertical overlap will need to be reduced drastically.
3. Angle Class III: incisors edge-to-edge and very occasionally in reverse overjet.

Setting up posterior teeth

In setting up the posterior teeth, the surgeon or technician should aim to place the teeth in the neutral zone and at the same time create a balanced articulation.

The definition of a balanced articulation is a continuous sliding contact of upper and lower cusps all round the dental arch during all closed grinding movements of the mandible.

The difference between a balanced articulation and a free articulation (p. 87) is that although there are free sliding movements with the lattter, balancing tooth contacts are not necessarily present on the side opposite to the occluding side.

To obtain a balanced articulation, teeth must be balanced for protrusive movements, then for lateral movements.

Factors in obtaining balanced protrusion

The theoretical factors in obtaining a balanced protrusion (Hanau's quint) are:

1. Condylar guidance.
2. Incisal guidance.
3. Cusp angle of posterior teeth.
4. Orientation of occlusal plane.
5. Prominence of compensating curve.

These factors are interdependent and when one factor is changed alteration is required in some, or all, of the others to maintain a state of balance.

Condylar guidance

This is the only factor fixed by the patient. It should not be changed. An average value for the condylar guidance angle is 30°.

Incisal guidance

Incisal guidance is the angle at which the lower incisor slides down the palatal surface of the upper. It is set according to the relationships of the upper and lower incisors.

As stated previously, the incisive guidance table is usually set at an angle between 10° and 20°. Most clinicians start with the table angulated at 10° and only increase it if a deep overbite is required for aesthetic reasons. Furthermore most clinicians are reluctant to increase the angle beyond 20° because, to compensate for this, either steep cusp angles, a steeply inclined occlusal plane, or a compensating curve of short radius must be used (3,4 and 5 of Hanau's quint). All these compensations are unfavourable to satisfactory complete denture construction.

Cusp angle on posterior teeth

This is chosen by the prosthetist. Steep cusp angles (30–40°) are chosen where a steep incisal guidance is necessary. Generally cusp angles of 0–20° are most satisfactory.

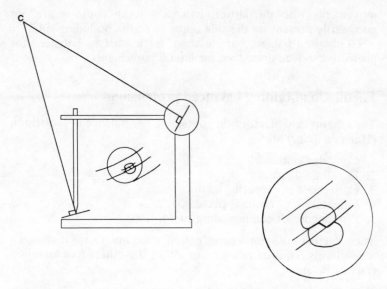

Figure 19.5 Balance in protrusion in theory. In protrusion the teeth should move along arcs whose centre is C

In theory only, the cuspal angle required to obtain balance in protrusion is obtained as follows (Figure 19.5). Right angle projections are taken from the centre of the incisal guidance table and from the condylar track. These two projections will intersect at a point above the articulator. From this intersection curves are traced through the occlusal plane. Teeth with cusp angles conforming to these curves will be balanced in protrusion. The contact path of anterior teeth should also conform to these curves.

The orientation of the occlusal plane

The orientation of the occlusal plane in an anteroposterior direction is determined at the occlusal registration stage provided a facebow is used. Slight alterations are acceptable at the set-up stage.

The compensating curve

This indicates how the molars diverge from the general occlusal plane (Figure 19.6). It is necessary to prevent excessively steep posterior cusp angles.

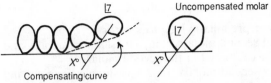

Figure 19.6 Compensating curve reducing cuspal angles. |7 which has been compensated (on left) has shallower cusps than the uncompensated |7, yet the angle of the cusps to the horizontal plane ($x°$) is the same in both

Lateral balance

During lateral excursions the movements of the condyles differ. The working side condyle remains in the glenoid fossa, while the balance side condyle moves down the articular eminence. The angle through which the molar teeth move is primarily affected by the condylar angle, and the angle through which the anterior teeth move by the incisive guidance angle. Thus, on the working side where the condyle only rotates slightly, the posterior teeth move through a nearly horizontal path (i.e. about 3°) and the anterior teeth move through an angle approaching 10°. On the balancing side the posterior teeth move through a path which approaches the condylar angle (i.e. about 20° if the condylar angle is 30°) and the anterior teeth through an angle which approaches 10°.

In order to balance the teeth during these lateral excursions, the upper teeth must be inclined buccally to create a lateral compensating curve similar to that described by Monson for the natural dentition. Figure 19.7 is a complex diagram which shows the relationship between this compensating curve and the ideal cuspal angles for balance during working and balancing movements.

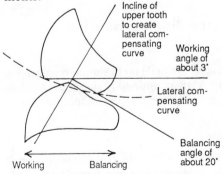

Figure 19.7 Diagram to show interrelationship during lateral movements between cuspal angles and compensating curve

The posterior teeth are set up as follows:

1. Upper and lower premolars: long axis vertical.
2. Upper first and second molars: long axis sloping buccally and distally. More accentuated in the second molars.
3. Lower first and second molars: long axis sloping lingually and mesially to occlude with upper teeth.

The fallacy of cuspal angles

Prosthetic textbooks are filled with diagrams of cuspal angles and their relationship to paths of movement. However many diagrams are incorrect since cusps do not move on the surface of one another. They usually move along fissure patterns. Thus the mesiopalatal cusp of the upper first molar occludes with the central fossa of the lower molar. It moves long the mesiodistal fissure during protrusion and along the buccolingual fissure during lateral movements (Figure 19.8).

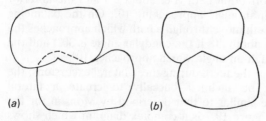

(a)   (b)

Figure 19.8 (a) demonstrates the actual molar relationship in the mouth; (b) the incorrect relationship as shown in some textbooks

The setting up of teeth according to anatomical landmarks

As has been stressed previously, artificial teeth should be placed in the neutral zone to help attain optimum stability. Certain anatomical landmarks aid in the correct setting of teeth.

Incisal papilla and upper incisors

If the contact point between the central incisors is placed 10 mm in front of the mid point of the incisal papilla, the incisors are likely to be near their pre-extraction position (Figure 19.9).

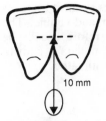

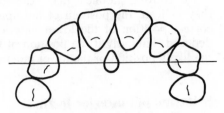

Figure 19.9 The relationship between the incisors and the incisal papilla

Figure 19.10 Line through incisal papilla passes through canines

Incisal papilla and upper canines

If a line through the centre of the canines passes near the posterior border of the incisal papilla, the canines are likely to be near their correct position (Figure 19.10).

Remnant of linguogingival margin and upper molars

When the upper molars are extracted, a fine scar or cordlike elevation may be seen running near the crest of the alveolus. It represents the former junction of the palatal gingiva with the teeth and is the remnant of the linguogingival margin. Watt (1960) studied this scar using tattoos before and after extraction. He showed that this scar moves about 3 mm buccally over a period of several years, due to underlying alveolar bone resorption. Setting molar teeth with a 3 mm overlap on the scar places them near their pre-extraction position (Figure 19.11).

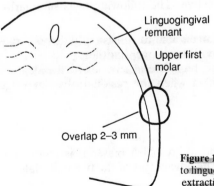

Linguogingival
remnant

Upper first
molar

Overlap 2–3 mm

Figure 19.11 Relation of upper first molar to linguogingival scar a few years after extraction

The above anatomical guides can on occasions be most useful as they indicate the position of the upper incisor and canine. The correct position of the lower anterior can therefore usually be deduced. Similarly if the position of the upper molars is known, the likely position of the lower molars can be estimated.

Selection of posterior teeth

Posterior teeth are selected primarily for their efficiency in mastication. The main variables are:

1. Width of teeth.
2. Anatomical or non-anatomical teeth.
3. Acrylic or porcelain.

Width of posterior teeth

Generally posterior teeth which are narrow buccolingually are better than those of a standard width. Narrow posterior teeth allow food to be triturated with less force. This reduces the load transmitted to the residual ridge and allows for more favourable contouring of the polished surfaces of the dentures.

Anatomical or non-anatomical teeth

Anatomical teeth are those that are shaped like a conventional tooth with cusps and fissures. Non-anatomical teeth come in a wide range of designs including flat plane teeth (also called flat cusp), teeth with metal inserts (e.g. Sosins–Levin), and inverted cusp teeth with hollows in the occlusal surface (e.g. Halls teeth).

Clinicians are divided in their opinion as to which design of posterior tooth is most effective. The following facts summarize the situation:

1. No clinical studies have been able to consistently demonstrate the superiority of one tooth form over another.
2. High cusp teeth transmit high lateral stresses to the denture base and are best avoided when the residual alveolar ridge shows marked atrophy.

Acrylic or porcelain

Again clinicians are divided as to which material is considered better for posterior teeth. The advantages of the two materials are discussed in Chapter 6, p. 38.

Phonetics

Many patients complain of phonetic problems when first receiving complete dentures. Fortunately most of these problems resolve within a few days as the patient adapts to the new shape within their mouth. Longstanding speech problems can be difficult to resolve. Difficulties usually occur with consonant sounds which are formed in six main mouth positions (Table 19.1).

Table 19.1 Mouth positions for some English consonants

Mouth position	Description of position	Consonant
Lingual dental	Tip of tongue on upper anterior teeth	'th'
Anterior lingual palatal	Tip of tongue on anterior part of palate	's', 'ch', 'j'
Posterior lingual palatal	Tongue on posterior of hard palate	'k'
Lateral linguodental	Side of tongue on palate	'l'
Labial	Lips brought together and separated suddenly	'b', 'p'
	Lips brought together and separated slowly	'm'
Labiodental	Lower lip inside upper anterior teeth	'f', 'v'

When there are difficulties with phonetics, the operator should ascertain which consonants are faulty. It is likely that one particular mouth position is involved. Alterations to the dentures should then be directed at regions in that specific mouth position. For example, the most common problem is lisping where 's' sounds as 'th'. The consonant 's' is formed in the anterior lingual palatal position, the tongue forming a channel with the palate. To correct lisping it must be possible for the patient to form this tongue channel. This may be done by thinning the palate anteriorly, widening the arch in the canine region, or moving the upper anterior teeth forward.

Chapter 20

Aesthetics and trial insertion

Most dentists try and make dentures that look as natural as possible. Many patients, however, want to look as young as possible and ask for small white teeth in a vain attempt to recapture a lost youth. How much the surgeon should enforce his views concerning aesthetics on the patient is controversial. What, for instance, is the correct dental appearance for a middle-aged lady with blue hair, green eye-shadow, bright red lips and purple glitter spectacle frames? In many cases a compromise has to be reached. This chapter describes the factors which contribute to the natural appearance of the teeth and associated structures.

Factors involved in aesthetics

The factors involved in aesthetics are:
1. Denture base – must be stable and retentive.
2. General position of teeth.
3. Vertical dimension.
4. The selection of colour.
5. The selection of size.
6. The selection of tooth shape.
7. The selection of tooth material.
8. The arrangement of individual teeth.

Denture base

The denture base must be stable and retentive, otherwise all attempts at realism are immediately lost. If the patient shows any gumwork on smiling or laughing, the colour, shape and extent of the base must be considered carefully.

General position of teeth

Teeth erupt into the neutral zone which is the resultant of the lingual and buccal forces acting on them. When the teeth are removed a potential space remains, i.e. the denture space.

The aim is to place the artificial teeth in the same position as their natural predecessors. Patients with marked protrusion of the anterior teeth may ask for this to be reduced. However, if this is done a feeling of discomfort and instability of the dentures may result. Nevertheless, the patient will often tolerate this because of the improved aesthetics.

Vertical dimension

For good aesthetics the occlusal vertical dimension must be correct. If it is too great, the patient may complain of a mouth full of teeth with a stretched facial appearance. If the vertical dimension is too small, the patient will have the typical overclosed appearance shown in Figure 2.3.

The selection of anterior teeth for colour

A tooth is basically yellow with red, grey, blue or brown tinting. Teeth darken with age. By and large, artificial teeth should be matched to the colour that the natural ones would have been, were they still present.

Any single tooth may have a gradation of colour with translucency of the incisal edge and a darkening towards the neck. Individual teeth within the arch also vary. The central incisors are often lighter than the laterals and the canines darker still.

Brown vertical cracks can often be seen in the incisors of the elderly; accordingly one manufacturer incorporates this feature in some anterior teeth. Cervical staining may also be marked. Furthermore, brown bars of dentine may be visible when the enamel is worn away, especially in the lower incisors. All these features can be reproduced in acrylic teeth using proprietary stains (Figure 20.1).

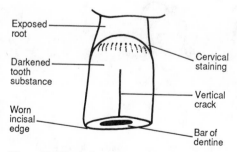

Exposed root

Darkened tooth substance

Worn incisal edge

Cervical staining

Vertical crack

Bar of dentine

Figure 20.1 Typical age changes seen in a tooth

The selection of anterior teeth for size

The width of the teeth is usually in proportion to that of the patient's head. Prominent canine eminences are still present in many edentulous patients. Measuring the distance between the distal surfaces of these two prominences gives a good indication of the width of the six upper anterior teeth (Figure 20.2).

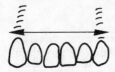

Figure 20.2 Distance between canine eminences indicating width of upper anterior teeth

Some clinicians consider that the width of the subject's nose corresponds to the distance between the tips of the upper canines.

Anthropometric studies have shown that the bizygomatic width divided by 3.3 gives an indication of the combined width of the upper six anterior teeth. Dividing the bizygomatic width by 16 gives an indication of the width of one upper central incisor. (Bizygomatic width is the greatest distance between the zygomatic arch of each side of the face.)

The selection of anterior teeth for shape

In 1914 Leon Williams classified tooth forms according to the inverted shape of the face below the forehead (Figure 20.3). He described square, ovoid and tapering types. This system has been widely adopted and used by practitioners, but several studies have shown that no such relationship exists.

Irrespective of the shape which is chosen, the proportion of the width to the height is most important in order to achieve satisfactory cosmetic results. The length should be between 1.25 and 1.5 the dimension of the width.

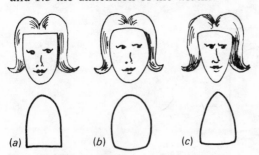

Figure 20.3 The supposed relationship between face form and tooth shape: (a) square; (b) ovoid; (c) tapering

The shape of a tooth can change with age, following incisal attrition and gingival recession. For instance, a rounded tooth may become squarer as the incisal edge is worn away and longer as gum recession occurs.

The selection of material

Quality acrylic teeth have as good an appearance as porcelain. However, appearance may deteriorate with both materials, for acrylic suffers from abrasive wear, and porcelain may chip.

Arrangement of individual teeth

For a good aesthetic result, the following guidelines should be noted:

1. Centre line of face coincident with centre line of arch.
2. The canines are the turning point of the arch.
3. Facial asymmetry should be matched.
4. Position of teeth can be modified to promote individuality.

Irregularities can be created to give a natural appearance, e.g. diastemas, overlaps, crowding, etc. Perhaps one of the most effective ways of making the teeth look natural is to have an uneven 'sky line', i.e. the incisal edges of the teeth not all on the same plane (Figure 20.4).

The line of _321|123_ can be made to follow the line of the smiling lip to avoid a straight artificial appearance.

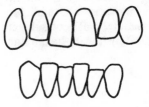

Figure 20.4 Irregular 'skyline' usually seen with natural teeth (look at your own)

Trial insertion

The object of this stage is to ensure that the dentures are satisfactory before processing in acrylic resin. The operator should methodically check all aspects of the denture as follows:

1. Outside the mouth: waxwork should be correctly contoured and extended into the sulci.

2. Singly in the mouth: there should be correct extension of the bases and stability should be satisfactory.
3. Together in the mouth: the following checks should be made:
   (a) Vertical dimension.
   (b) Occlusion.
   (c) Aesthetics. There should be correct lip support, and the appearance of the teeth should be natural. The correct position of the upper incisors can often be verified by phonetic tests. When pronouncing 'f' and 'v', the lower lip should just contact the upper incisal edges.
4. Patient's opinion: the patient is asked to look at the teeth in a hand mirror and asked for comments. Any necessary alterations are discussed and carried out when agreement is reached; a further appointment for a retry may be required.

The dentist should emphasize that any modifications must be carried out at this stage, as alterations to the processed denture are difficult and expensive. Fastidious or hesitant patients may be asked to sign a slip saying that the appearance of the teeth is satisfactory.

Post-dam (or posterior palatal seal)

The post-dam is placed along the posterior border of an upper complete denture about 1 mm anterior to the vibrating line. It should extend through the hamular notch just into the buccal sulcus. It may be produced by scraping the stone cast after the try-in stage (Figure 20.5). Most clinicians position it slightly anterior to the fovea palatina. In approximately 80% of subjects this corresponds to the position of the vibrating line in the midline.

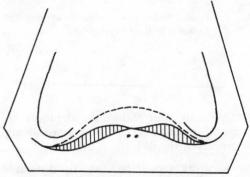

Figure 20.5 Shape of post-dam and position of anterior dam (if used)

The depth of the post-dam is approximately 1 mm, but it is slightly less in the midline where the tissues are barely displaceable.

Many clinicians cut the post-dam into the shape of a cupid's bow, chamfering it anteriorly into the displaceable mucosa. A second post-dam may be cut about 5 mm anterior to the first. It is claimed this second dam helps retain the thick mucous secretion from the posterior part of the palate, and so aids the posterior border seal.

Alternatively, a functional post-dam impression may be taken by adding greenstick composition to a permanent base and processing the addition in self-curing resin.

Chapter 21

Insertion of complete dentures

When inserting complete dentures, the operator should carefully check all features of the new prosthesis. However carefully dentures are made, minor modifications are frequently necessary at this stage. This is primarily due to shrinkage which occurs during the polymerization of poly(methyl methacrylate).

Checks before inserting dentures

Before inserting the dentures, check the following:

1. Fitting surface: look and feel for pimples of acrylic resin and remove if necessary.
2. Polished surface: should be checked for roughness.
3. Periphery: this should be rounded except in the posterior border of the upper denture.
4. Occlusion: place dentures together by hand in maximum intercuspation. Check that the occlusal surfaces contact each other evenly; this simple test may reveal large errors in occlusion.

Inserting the upper denture

Firstly the upper denture only is inserted and a check of the following made:

1. Retention.
2. Stability.
3. Extension.
4. Undercuts.
5. Aesthetics.

Retention

Retention is checked by trying to remove the denture in an occlusal direction. If retention if poor it may be due to incorrect sulcus extension or width. Forward pressure applied to the upper incisors will tip the posterior edge of the denture down. If this occurs too readily the post-dam is defective or the extension of the denture into the hamular notch insufficient. Corrections should be made in greenstick or some similar material and then processed in self-curing acrylic resin.

Stability

Stability is checked by applying finger pressure to the occlusal surface. Force is then applied to alternate sides of the arch. If the denture moves with this test two possible faults may be present:

1. The posterior teeth have been set too far lateral to the alveolar ridge.
2. The shape and width of the flanges are insufficient to stabilize the denture (Figure 21.1).

Oral mucosa

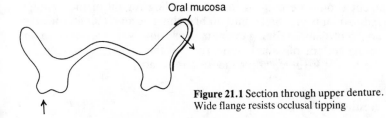

Figure 21.1 Section through upper denture. Wide flange resists occlusal tipping

If movements of the patient's mouth disturb the denture, the flange in the offending region should be adjusted for extension or width. This is a difficult task.

Extension

Extension of dentures should be checked. It is difficult to check over- or under-extension visually; on lifting the cheek to view the sulcus, the position and shape changes. Over-extended dentures tend to be unretentive and recoil when seated, and can be corrected with the aid of a disclosing agent. Under-extended dentures may be unretentive. The flange may be corrected with greenstick composition or a similar material, and the denture processed so the deficiency is made good with self-curing resin.

The periphery of the upper denture should also be checked to ensure that it extends correctly round the maxillary tuberosity into the hamular notch. The posterior border should lie just anterior to the vibrating line.

Undercuts

Edentulous models should be surveyed and undercuts blocked out. However, small undercuts may have been left intentionally on the denture to aid retention. If the alveolar mucosa is thick a slightly undercut denture flange may displace the tissue without pain. If, however, the mucosa is thin, it may not be possible to insert the denture. A disclosing agent such as pressure relief cream or disclosing wax should be applied to the periphery; an attempt should be made to seat the denture. The acrylic resin is relieved where the cream has been displaced. This is repeated until no indicator paste is dislodged and the denture can be inserted painlessly.

After the dentures have been fully seated areas of mucosal blanching should be sought. If these are found, again a disclosing agent should be applied to the offending region of the denture. Adjustments are made until no blanching occurs. (Many clinicians apply pressure relief cream or disclosing wax routinely to the fitting surface of complete dentures at this stage. They claim that the need for future adjustments is reduced.)

Aesthetics

Check that the appearance is satisfactory.

Inserting the lower denture

The same checks are made as for the upper denture:

1. Retention: it is hardly ever possible to obtain good retention with a complete lower denture.
2. Stability.
3. Extension: check especially that the posterior border covers at least one-third of the retromolar pad.
4. Undercuts: less likely on a lower complete denture.
5. Aesthetics.

Checking both dentures together

Finally, with both dentures in the mouth a check is made of:

1. Occlusion.
2. Vertical dimension.
3. Aesthetics.

Occlusion

The occlusion is checked first. RCP should coincide with PMI, i.e. when the patient occludes in RCP the dentures do not move. There should also be good balance of the arches in lateral and protrusive excursions.

The free-way space should be 2–4 mm unless otherwise planned. It is claimed that processing reduces the free-way space by 0.5–1 mm.

Precentric records
These are taken when dentures are to be remounted on an articulator. The patient is encouraged to bite into a softened horseshoe of wax in their most unstrained retruded position (i.e. RCP). The opposing cusps should be separated by about 1 mm of wax. If opposing cusps contact, deflective movements of one denture may occur; if so, the wax record should be repeated. Ideally a facebow record is also taken at this stage.

Adjusting the occlusion
Adjusting the occlusion of dentures at the insertion stage may be done in three ways:

1. By mounting the complete dentures, before insertion, back on the articulator on which they were originally set-up.
2. By taking a precentric record after insertion, and remounting the dentures on an articulator.
3. In the mouth using articulating paper or occlusal indicating paste.

The same procedure for adjusting the occlusion is followed whether the dentures are adjusted on an articulator or in the mouth. These are:

1. Occlude dentures in RCP. Record the occlusion with articulating paper. There should be an even distribution of marks around the arch. If not, grind the fossae until there is even contact.

2. Move articulator arm into lateral excursion. Grind the cusps to relieve interfering contacts on working and balancing side. Repeat on the other side.
3. Slide the denture into protrusion. Grind lower incisal edges if there is interference.

When the occlusal adjustments are complete, polish acrylic teeth with pumice or polish porcelain teeth with rubber-bonded abrasive wheels followed by pumice.

Vertical dimension

The BULL rule
When denture teeth are in RCP, the vertical dimension is maintained by the contact of the lower buccal cusps with the upper palatal cusps, except in cases of crossbite where the upper and lower cusp positions are reversed (Figure 21.2). If the vertical dimension is to be maintained these cusps should not be ground if

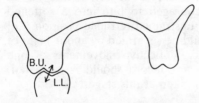

Figure 21.2 Section through upper denture. Grinding buccal upper (B.U.) and lingual lower (L.L.) cusps does not affect occlusal vertical dimension

possible. Note: sometimes grinding the 'forbidden cusps' is unavoidable, e.g. correcting a premature contact in the balancing lateral movement. Only the *B*uccal *U*pper and *L*ower *L*ingual cusps should be adjusted. (Some clinicians consider that the small change in vertical dimension incurred when adjusting all cusps on complete dentures is irrelevant, i.e. they believe the BULL rule lives up to its name!)

Advice to patients

Verbal advice to patients on the care of their dentures is best backed up by written instructions. An example of a patient advice sheet is shown in Figure 21.3.

Care of your dentures

Dentures are expensive. If you look after them well they will last longer, look better, and be more comfortable.

1. *If your dentures hurt* take them out and leave in water. Make an appointment to see your dentist. Wear them for a few hours before going to your dentist so he can see where they are rubbing.
2. *Eating and speaking* may be difficult at first. It will take a week or two to get used to your dentures. Cut your food into small pieces. Tough and sticky food can be particularly tricky.
3. *Clean* your dentures twice a day with a soft nail brush using soap and water. Clean them over a bowl of water so that if they drop they do not break. Alternatively, you may use a denture cleaner bought at a chemist.
4. *Keep* your dentures in water when not using them. This stops them warping.
5. *Night.* If you wear your dentures at night leave them out for an hour in the day to let your gums rest. Soak your dentures in water and use dilute bleach – about a teaspoonful to a glass of water – once a week, to disinfect the dentures.
6. *Check up.* You should return to your dentist in .... to check your dentures are still fitting properly and not harming your mouth.

Figure 21.3 Sample sheet: Care of your dentures

Notes on patient advice

The advice to patients wearing complete dentures is similar to that for patients wearing partial dentures (see p. 81).

If dentures are hurting, the patient should not persevere too much as this can lead to ulceration and delayed healing.

Patients who have not previously worn dentures sometimes expect too much from them, especially for ease of mastication and retention of the lower denture.

It is controversial whether dentures should be worn at night or not. If dentures are worn at night a slightly higher level of candidial infection (denture sore mouth) is found. Soaking the denture in an antifungal solution, i.e. dilute bleach, will prevent this. If dentures are not worn at night, it is claimed that the incidence of temporomandibular joint problems is greater. You can't win!

In point (6) on the advice sheet the surgeon fills in the recall date. If considerable bone resorption is anticipated, the patient is advised to return in six months. For other patients, approximately two years is recommended.

Denture cleansers

Soft debris and plaque can usually be removed from a denture with brushing. The hard deposits of calculus that adhere to a denture can be more difficult to remove. Ideally the patient should clean his/her dentures so that no plaque remains to subsequently be calcified.

There is a wide range of proprietary denture cleansers on the market. These are summarized in Table 21.1.

Table 21.1 Proprietary denture cleansers

Cleanser	Main constituent	Comments
Abrasives, either paste or powder	Abrasives such as calcium carbonate or plastic beads	Some brands abrade acrylic
Dilute acids	3–5% hydrochloric acid or sulphamic acid	Softens calculus. Brushing required after use
Oxygenating cleansers	Sodium perborate or percarbonate with an alkaline detergent	Most widely used cleansers. Bubbles remove debris. Not very effective since do not remove plaque
Hypochlorite solutions	Sodium hypochlorite (bleach)	Effective at removing plaque and heavy stain. Prolonged use may corrode cobalt-chromium
Enzyme cleansers	Proteolytic enzymes	Not widely available

Chapter 22

Special techniques for complete dentures

Palateless dentures

These are constructed for patients who persistently retch with conventional complete upper dentures. Retching in denture wearers is usually triggered by contact of the denture with the tongue or hard palate. Some patients are unable to tolerate the contact of a denture with the posterior two-thirds of the hard palate. In these cases, a palateless denture is often the only tolerable appliance, but the retention is frequently poor. This can sometimes be improved by using a wide rolled border, obtained with a composition impression. Furthermore, with such a material the impression can quickly be removed from the mouth if the patient experiences discomfort. Some operators like the technician to produce a dam around the entire periphery of the denture; this is known as a food line.

Microvalves are sometimes used in such dentures. At first they are effective but soon become useless as the valve clogs with food debris.

Training bases

A few patients are not able to wear and use conventional complete dentures. They are often those who have been edentulous for years and never worn a denture. When these patients are fitted with complete dentures they are unable to control them. Chronic retchers may also be helped with training bases.

A training base is a plastic base-plate covering the denture-bearing area of the mouth (Figure 22.1). Usually such bases are constructed for both the upper and lower edentulous ridges. Most

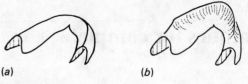

Figure 22.1 (*a*) Lower training base. (*b*) The training base after application of tissue conditioning material

patients are able to tolerate wearing just these plates initially. Gradually over a period of weeks the training bases are built up occlusally with a material such as cold-curing acrylic resin or tissue conditioner. When a reasonable vertical dimension is reached, usually after several weeks, acrylic teeth are substituted to form a conventional denture.

Techniques for loose lower dentures

The loose lower complete denture is one of the most common problems in prosthetic dentistry. Many methods have been developed over the years to try and combat this problem. Some are described below.

Neutral zone techniques

The importance of the neutral zone has been described previously. A number of techniques have been described to establish the neutral zone using impression materials, e.g. tissue conditioner has been used, placed occlusally on acrylic bases. This is gradually built up over a period of hours – sometimes days – and is moulded by the surrounding muscles into the neutral zone. In another technique wax occlusal rims are cut away in selected regions and substituted by alginate impression material; this is moulded into the neutral zone as it sets. In both techniques, artificial teeth are subsequently set in the position of the neutral zone.

Anthropoidal pouch technique

The buccinator has a natural pouch immediately anterior to the masseter. (You can feel it with your own finger. Monkeys have a well developed pouch here where they are able to store food.) This pouch can be utilized to stabilize lower dentures by extending the buccal surface into it.

Essentially the technique involves adding impression material (alginate or zinc oxide/eugenol) onto the buccal surface of the lower complete denture. This is carried out at the trial insertion stage. In the original description of the technique, a special tray with vertical walls in the molar region was used and an impression of the fitting, buccal and lingual surfaces taken simultaneously (Figure 22.2). (With this particular technique the position of the neutral zone is also found.)

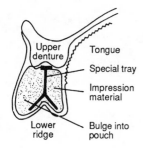

Figure 22.2 Diagram of anthropoidal pouch technique. Coronal section through molar region. In this case a special tray with vertical walls is being used to record the pouch

Impression material about the size of a walnut is usually formed from the anthropoidal pouch. This bulge is reproduced in the completed dentures.

The lingual pouch technique

This was first described by Sir Wilfred Fish. In this technique the posterior lingual flange of a lower complete denture was extended medially under the base of the tongue. The object was to create a stable denture, retained by the base of the tongue.

This technique can be effective, but the large flanges are often not tolerated by the patient. Moreover it may be necessary to reduce a sharp mylohyoid ridge surgically in order to gain access to the posterolingual area.

Weighted complete lower dentures

These were popular some decades ago, and used in the belief that this would improve the retention and stability. The denture was weighted by incorporating a silver or similar alloy which, because of its dark appearance, was placed as a reline material adjacent to the oral mucosa.

Springs

Springs were once a popular method of stabilizing lower complete dentures. These were attached to both upper and lower dentures in the molar area of the buccal flange. They worked by forcing the dentures apart, and so stabilizing the lower denture against the lower alveolus. Although fairly successful, they unfortunately constituted a food trap. They are sometimes used today for obturators.

Chapter 23

The damage dentures can cause

This chapter considers the damage that dentures can cause to the surrounding tissues other than the teeth and gingiva. Most of these conditions are common but irreversible damage can occur if they are not treated.

Injuries to the mouth from dentures may be either acute or chronic:

1. Acute conditions: occurring within a short period after the denture is fitted and usually painful.
2. Chronic conditions: occurring over a long period and not necessarily painful.

Acute conditions

Signs and symptoms commonly found are:

1. Pain.
2. Redness, possibly with oedema.
3. Ulceration of the mucosa, usually with a yellow sloughing base.
4. Ulceration of the cheek along the occlusal line, due to cheek biting.

Acute damage due to complete dentures may be caused by the following:

1. Errors in base extension: over-extension, rarely under-extension.
2. Discrepancies in the fit surface which have been missed.
3. Errors in recording RCP.
4. Incorrectly shaped polished surface.
5. Teeth set in wrong position.
6. Vertical dimension too great.
7. Lateral and protrusive contacts not balanced.

In addition to the above, the partial denture may also cause acute damage by:

1. Clasps engaging too deep an undercut causing periodontitis.
2. Rests placed on weak restorations causing fracture of the same.
3. Major or minor connectors interfering with muscle activity.
4. Poorly supported dentures physically damaging mucosa.
5. Allergy to constituent of denture, e.g. nickel.

Chronic conditions

When the patient does not attend for aftercare, chronic damage may be caused to the oral tissues.

Complete dentures

Due to resorption, the denture base may cease to fit the edentulous ridge. This may cause:

1. Increased resorption.
2. Production of bony or soft tissue abnormalities.
3. Hyperplasia of the oral mucosa.
4. Denture stomatitis.
5. Hyperkeratosis.

Partial dentures

In addition to the above, partial dentures may also cause the following chronic damage:

1. Damage to abutment tooth leading to fracture or loss.
2. Damage to restorations.
3. Stripping of gingiva.
4. Temporomandibular joint symptoms – usually due to a faulty occlusion.
5. Badly designed denture causing food stagnation.

Edentulous patients often feel that regular visits to the dentist are no longer necessary except for major problems such as fracture. Unfortunately this may be aggravated by the dental surgeon and his staff who do not caution patients that regular review visits are necessary for inspection and maintenance of their dentures. Routine aftercare for the denture patient does not appear to be practised.

The authors consider that complete denture patients should be advised to have a '3000 meal' service every two years!

Reasons for denture patients seeking treatment

Where there is no recall system, complete denture patients generally seek advice for one of four reasons:

1. Fracture of denture.
2. Pain.
3. Impaired function.
4. Changes in appearance.

Fracture of the denture

Fracture of the denture or loss of denture teeth is the most common cause of patients seeking help.

Pain

Pain or inability to wear the dentures is usually due to instability and lack of retention of the base, due to changes in the supporting tissues. Problems related to resorption of the basal support tissue depend upon the type of denture prescribed. Inevitably, the relining of immediate dentures is required soon after insertion. This period varies according to the number and position of extracted teeth but should not exceed six months. However, all too often patients persist in wearing immediate dentures long after adjustment is required; this may cause severe damage to the supporting tissue.

Impaired function

Mastication, swallowing and speech can all be adversely affected by reduced retention and stability. This may also be caused by wear of the material – almost always acrylic – from which the dentures are constructed. In addition the patient may adopt an abnormal – usually protrusive – posture because of the occlusal wear.

Changes in appearance

The patient may seek advice where the appearance of the denture is adversely affected due to loss of teeth, wear or staining.

Loss of occlusal face height may lead to changes in the patient's appearance leading to the familiar overclosed facial contour. Although the patient may feel that the dentures are still generally comfortable, comments by the patient's relatives may prompt a visit to the surgery.

Consequence of lack of aftercare for complete dentures

Lack of aftercare may have the following consequences:

1. Damage to supporting tissues.
2. Alteration to facial musculature.
3. Pathology of oral tissues.

Damage to supporting tissues

This usually involves the mucoperiosteum and underlying bone; it may be localized or generalized and may or may not give rise to pain.

Alteration of the facial musculature and damage to the temporomandibular joints

This may appear as peculiar posturing, or the development of a habit after long-term wear of dentures which have outlived their useful life.

Pathology

Since dentures are provided for the more elderly patients it would seem logical to review the oral tissues of these patients on a regular, possibly annual, basis. In this way not only can the dentures be properly maintained but the oral tissues can be examined for early signs of pathology; this may or may not be associated with the wearing of dentures. Lesions such as denture stomatitis, or rarely neoplasia, can thus be diagnosed and treated in good time.

Denture stomatitis

This is incorrectly termed denture sore mouth as no pain or soreness is manifest with the condition. It is usually caused by *Candida albicans* although occasionally other *Candida* species may be present. The palate is red, sometimes with petechial and whitish areas, which are evidence of active candidial colonies.

For confirmation of the initial diagnosis, the following may be sent for pathological examination:

1. A 5 ml saliva sample.
2. A scraping from an area beneath the dentures.

3. In some cases, the denture itself for use in an imprint culture.
4. Blood for haematological examination, if a systemic pathology is suspected.

The material provided is cultured on Saboraud's corn meal agar. High counts of *Candida* organisms and the presence of hyphae confirm the diagnosis.

Treatment of denture stomatitis

1. Instruct the patient to leave the denture out at night and soak it in Milton or dilute bleach (both hypochlorities) which are antifungal. This treatment is effective since denture stomatitis is often (if not always) caused by colonies of *Candida* growing on the fitting surface of the denture itself.
2. Antifungal therapy using nystatin lozenges, amphotericin, or miconazole.
3. Review the patient at regular intervals.
4. Remake the dentures if necessary.

Angular cheilitis

This is seen as red or ulcerated areas on the corner of the mouth and may also be present. It is usually due to seepage of infected saliva at the corners of the mouth. It is treated in a manner similar to denture stomatitis, namely:

1. Soak dentures in hypochlorite.
2. Apply antifungal creams to infected area.
3. Remake dentures if necessary. Note: overclosure of dentures will exaggerate the creases at the angle of the mouth.

Angular cheilitis and oral candidiasis may be a reflection of systemic disease (e.g. iron deficiency anaemia) which should be treated with the cooperation of the patient's physician. Rarely the infection may be streptococcal. Cases not responding to treatment may therefore require bacteriological analysis.

Relining

Relining consists of adding denture base material to the fitting surface of a denture to improve its adaptation to the tissues. Relining complete dentures is done to improve retention and stability. It is necessary because resorption of alveolar bone causes the accuracy of fit of complete dentures to deteriorate. Dentures may be considered for relining if:

1. The vertical dimension is satisfactory.
2. The occlusal surfaces have not worn smooth.
3. The dentures are generally satisfactory with regard to aesthetics, base extension, RCP, etc.

Clinical procedure

1. Clean fitting surface of denture.
2. Remove all undercuts. (If this is not done the rigid plastic may not be able to be removed from the stone casts after the reline has been cast.)
3. Shorten flanges by 1 mm so there is no danger of over-extension.
4. Minor defects or base extension can be corrected with green-stick impression compound.
5. Take an impression within the dentures using a suitable impression material (usually zinc oxide/eugenol).
6. Impressions should be taken within upper and lower dentures together, with the patient occluding in RCP.
7. Cast impressions in stone.
8. Flask dentures still on stone cast in a manner similar to that used for flasking wax dentures.
9. Separate flasks.
10. Remove dentures from stone casts. Remove impression material thoroughly and process acrylic resin on to impression surface of denture.

Rebasing

This is similar to relining except that the palate is cut out of an upper denture and replaced with one of orthodox thickness. It is necessary when relining would lead to an excessive thickness of acrylic in the palatal region of a denture; this commonly occurs when a denture is relined for the second time.

Section 4

Special denture prosthetics

Chapter 24

Obturators, overdentures and implants

Obturators

Obturators are only briefly described since they are relatively rare and most practitioners or students will never make one. Overdentures are discussed more fully since they are eminently suitable for construction in general practice.

Obturators are artificial devices for sealing a defect. Dental obturators, in addition to sealing a defect, usually replace teeth, alveolar bone, and adjacent missing structures such as parts of the maxilla.

Jaw bone may be lost and need replacement due to:

1. Surgery.
2. Trauma.
3. Developmental defects, especially cleft palate.
4. Infection, e.g. osteomyelitis.

If, for example, maxillary bone is lost, facial form and function are restored to a varying degree by attaching an obturator to an upper denture. This often consists of a hollow bulb of acrylic resin (Figure 24.1). Other plastic or rubber materials may be used, e.g. silicone-based rubbers, or polyvinyl chloride (PVC).

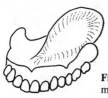

Figure 24.1 Typical obturator; hollow bulb of acrylic restores maxilla lost by surgery

Overdentures

Definition: Dentures which derive support from one or more abutment teeth by completely enclosing them beneath the fitting surface, i.e. dentures that cover the roots and utilize them for support (Figure 24.2).

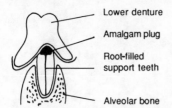

Lower denture

Amalgam plug

Root-filled support teeth

Alveolar bone

Figure 24.2 Typical overdenture: root-filled premolar supports lower complete denture. N.B. for clarity overdenture is shown separated from tissues and root face

The roots of teeth unsuitable for use as abutments for a removable partial denture may be employed. Loss of supporting bone causes the crown:root ratio to become increasingly unfavourable (Figure 24.3). Horizontal forces on the tooth are increasingly more damaging. A dramatic improvement in crown:root ratio is achieved by reducing the crowns to 1 or 2 mm above the gingival margin, which vastly reduces the lateral leverage on the remaining root.

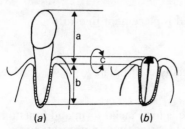

(a)   (b)

Figure 24.3 Change in crown:root ratio after preparing tooth as overdenture support: (*a*) crown:root ratio is a:b; (*b*) crown:root ratio is c:b

Overdentures may be complete or partial. For instance, with a partial overdenture a free-end saddle may be avoided by retaining a root-filled root of a lower second or third molar.

Advantages of overdentures

The advantages of overdentures derive principally from the retained roots and are as follows:

1. Preservation of remaining alveolar bone around the retained root.
2. Greater stability and retention of the denture.

3. Sensory feedback from periodontal membrane of retained root.
4. Greater masticatory force possible.
5. Retaining devices can be attached to remaining roots.
6. Reduction of psychological trauma for some patients.
7. If an abutment root is lost, additions to the denture are easy and inexpensive.

The sensory and proprioceptive feedback from the retained periodontal membrane is of importance. It probably aids the patient's recognition of:

1. Jaw position.
2. Food texture.
3. Muscle force used in mastication.

Research has shown that natural molars can discriminate a threshold load one-tenth of that detected by complete dentures.

The retained root may have various retaining devices attached to it by means of a post (Figure 24.4). These male attachments (patrices) join female counterparts (matrices) within the body of the denture and provide very positive retention. However these

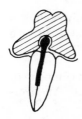

Figure 24.4 Diagram of post-retained attachment

devices are expensive and need frequent skilful maintenance. There may also be insufficient space to accommodate them in the denture and their bulk may obliterate the free-way space. Magnets are now also being used for retention of overdentures. They have the advantage of exerting less lateral force to the retained root.

Disadvantages of overdentures

1. More clinical time and expense.
2. Difficult time-consuming endodontics may be necessary.
3. Patient must have good oral hygiene or roots will be lost due to caries and periodontal disease.
4. Increased labial or buccal fullness around retained roots due to lack of resorption.

5. Increased masticatory load and often smaller inter-ridge distance may predipose to denture breakage. This problem can be helped by using high impact resins or metal alloys in the denture.
6. More frequent denture maintenance visits necessary.

Uses of overdentures

Overdentures are particularly useful for the following cases:

1. A complete denture opposed by natural teeth.
2. Cleft palates.
3. Hypodontia.
4. Extreme attrition.
5. Potentially difficult lower complete dentures.
6. Bruxists.

Patients with complete dentures opposing natural teeth can experience difficulty with dentures. The alignment of the occlusal plane can make occlusal balance difficult, but by making an overdenture this problem can be solved.

Extreme attrition is not rare. Patients are frequently seen who have worn their anterior teeth down often to gum level. In such cases crowning can be very difficult. Overdentures can be constructed with the minimum of tooth preparation.

Bruxists with conventional complete dentures often complain of widespread soreness over the denture-bearing area. An overdenture will often prevent this complaint developing.

Patient selection

With an overdenture, the patient must exercise special care in maintaining the health of the abutment teeth and of the gingival tissues. In selecting suitable patients, the following factors should be considered:

1. General health, e.g. heart valve disease, adversely affecting the prescription of endodontic treatment.
2. Cooperation of patient.
3. Attitude of patient, especially regarding tooth loss.
4. Oral hygiene.
5. Periodontal state of potential abutment.
6. Sufficient inter-ridge space (critical if attachments used).

Clinical procedure

The retained tooth is root-treated. If caries is unlikely to occur, the root face is prepared so that 2 mm projects from the gingival margin and the root face is left bare – apart from the restoration required to seal off the root canal filling. If caries is likely, a coping is necessary. This is a covering for the entire root surface and is usually made of cast gold (Figure 24.5). A coping is also required if caries has destroyed the root surface and it cannot be stoned so that 2 mm projects above the gingival margin.

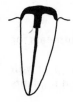

Figure 24.5 One form of gold coping

Often with an older patient the root will not need to be devitalized, since deposition of secondary dentine will allow sufficient preparation of the root face without exposing the pulp. In these patients the root face may be left intact after removal of sharp enamel projections. Copings may be fitted as required, but will need small pins (e.g. Williams) to aid retention.

Two clinical methods may be used in the construction of overdentures:

1. After the abutments have been prepared and stoned to gingival level, impressions are taken and dentures made using routine procedures.
2. The teeth are root-treated but not stoned to the level of the gingiva. The dentures are then constructed as for immediate replacements, the clinician having reduced the height of the prospective abutments on the master cast to about 4 mm above the gingiva. On completion of the dentures, the teeth are reduced in the mouth and the dentures fitted as accurately as possible. Cold-cured acrylic resin is then placed on the fitting surface of the denture in the recesses which correspond to the abutments, venting holes having been cut right through to the polished surface. When set the resin is trimmed away and the final fit of the dentures checked with disclosing paste. Finally the occlusion is perfected.

Denture maintenance

This should be as follows:

1. Abutments are examined at six-monthly intervals.
2. Patient is instructed to brush over abutments twice a day. Topical fluoride in the form of toothpaste should be applied once a day, using the denture as applicator.
3. Denture must be kept clean. An interspace brush may be used to clean the recesses on the fitting surface. The denture should not be worn at night.

Implants

Definition: An insert into the oral tissues to provide abutments for crowns, dentures or bridges.

Over the years many types of implant have been tried, most with only limited success; however, the latest osseointegrated implants do seem to show great promise.

Types of implant are:

1. Endosseous.
2. Subperiosteal.
3. Submucous.
4. Endodontic.
5. Augmentation.
6. Osseointegrated.

Endosseous

Endosseous implants involve part of the fixation system entering the jaw bone (Figure 24.6). The intra-osseous end may be a variety of shapes including screw, blade or pin. The dentures are retained

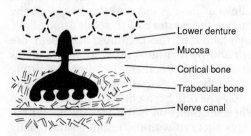

Figure 24.6 Diagram of blade implant in mandible

retained by a projection from the implant into the fitting surface of the denture. Endosseous implants have not proved to be successful due to infection tracking into the bone from the oral cavity.

Subperiosteal

Subperiosteal implants lie on the surface of bone beneath the mucoperiosteum and are retained by this tough fibrous layer. Highly polished vertical posts project through the mucosa and act as abutments for the denture (Figure 24.7). Clinically the mucoperiosteum is stripped back and an impression taken of the cortical surface of the bone. The implant is fitted some days later.

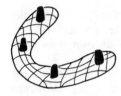

Figure 24.7 Subperiosteal implant; the framework rests upon the cortex and is retained by the mucoperiosteum. Posts project through the mucosa to retain the denture

These implants have proved more successful than endosseous implants, with many reports of a useful life of over 20 years. However, they also suffer the problem of infections tracking in from the oral cavity.

Submucous

A series of studs is attached to the fitting surface of the upper denture corresponding to that area of the palate which has a well developed submucosal layer. At the time of insertion of the denture, incisions are made in the epithelium to allow the studs to penetrate the wound. The epithelium eventually grows down to line the stud cavity.

This technique has not been successful as the pockets form an ideal nidus for bacterial growth; furthermore the pockets will close if the denture is left out for too long.

Endodontic

Root-filled teeth are transfixed by a pin which protrudes through the apex into the surrounding bones. These pins may be used for denture retention or to immobilize loose teeth.

Ridge augmentation

Attempts have been made to improve the height of the alveolar ridge by the insertion of various materials beneath the periosteum. Hydroxyapatite preparations have been used with some success, but difficulty is encountered in mobilizing enough periosteum.

Materials

The metals at present used for dental implants are titanium and alloys of cobalt-chromium and molybdenum, e.g. Vitallium, Coe-form, Wisil.

Shortcomings

The shortcomings of the above implants are:

1. When most needed they are contraindicated; for example, resorption in the mandible exposing the inferior alveolar canal, and in the upper jaw when the maxillary antrum is in close proximity to the alveolus.
2. As the implant has no epithelial attachment, unlike the attachment between enamel and the gingiva, infection can track into the subepithelial tissues.
3. With an endosseus implant, any load transmitted to the blade is transferred to cancellous bone. This is likely to resorb in response to this force.

Osseointegrated

Branemark and his colleagues in Sweden have spent 25 years researching the osseointegration system of implants. The basis of the technique is that if titanium (a pure metal and not an alloy) is placed within the jaws, bone will form an intimate relationship with it with no intervening fibrous tissue.

Very briefly, the technique for osseointegrated implants is as follows:

1. The site for the implants is anterior to the mental foramen in the lower jaw and anterior to the antra in the upper jaw.
2. A flap is raised and the jaw bone exposed.
3. Vertical channels 3.5 mm in width are cut into the bone. During cutting the temperature must not exceed 47°C. Very slow cutting speeds and copious water cooling are therefore used.
4. The implant is tapped into the bone. In shape it is a blind-ended tube. The open oral end is sealed with a domed screw. Up to five or six implants may be used per jaw.

5. The oral mucosa is sutured over the implant.
6. Two weeks after surgery the old denture, heavily eased, may be worn again.
7. Four to six months after the initial surgery the second phase is commenced. However, radiographs must show that osseointegration has taken place.
8. The top of the implants are surgically exposed and the sealing dome-shaped screw removed.
9. Copings are screwed into the centre of the implants to show their precise position and a very accurate impression of the jaws is taken.
10. Subsequently transmucosal abutments are screwed into the implants. They project several millimetres into the oral cavity.
11. A denture or bridge is able to unite the abutments. Its fitting surface contains small cylinders which precisely contain the abutments.

Note: The Branemark implant has, in effect, three portions: a blind-ended tube integrated within the jaw bone, a transmucosal abutment which screws into the implant and projects several millimetres into the oral cavity, and precise metal cylinders embedded into the fitting surface of the denture (or bridge) which marry up precisely with the transmucosal abutments.

Chapter 25

The problem denture patient

Complaints of complete denture wearers

Patients frequently require adjustments to even the most carefully made complete dentures. When the same patient returns for many adjustments they become a problem denture patient. It is extremely frustrating for a dental surgeon when a patient continually returns with various complaints, though the dentures appear satisfactory. An accurate diagnosis of the cause for complaint will save many hours of chairside time. In many cases the patient may have local, systemic or psychological problems which accentuate the difficulty.

The most common complaints are discussed below.

Pain under dentures

Pain under a specific area of recently fitted dentures is the most common complaint. A corresponding area of redness or an ulcer is usually seen in the mouth. When the operator has satisfied himself that there is no obvious cause of the pain – such as a wrongly recorded occlusion (see below) – the region of the denture fitting surface causing the pain should be reduced. The area of the denture to be adjusted is localized with the aid of a disclosing agent (e.g. disclosing wax or pressure-indicating paste) applied to the fitting surface of the denture. Such materials should be used with care as local oedema may increase the apparent area to be reduced, leading to a greater base reduction than is necessary. Denture fixative powder (whitened with zinc oxide) applied to the sore area will then adhere to the corresponding region of the denture when it is replaced. The denture may then be more accurately adjusted.

If the patient returns requesting more adjustments the surgeon should consider causes of trouble other than slight imperfections of the fitting surface. Such causes – most of which should have been spotted previously – include:

1. Incorrect recording of RCP or a poorly balanced articulation.
2. Absence of free-way space.
3. Retained root or other pathology.
4. Parafunctional conditions, e.g. bruxism.

When the occlusion is incorrect, the less retentive denture – usually the lower – moves slightly as opposing cusps interfere. Correction of this error is done by grinding, resetting the teeth, or remaking the dentures, depending on the severity of the problem. If the articulation is not balanced, either the occlusion will be locked and the patient will be unable to slide the dentures over one another, or the dentures will tip and move during masticatory movements.

When there is no free-way space, the patient usually complains of generalized soreness or pain over the whole denture-bearing area.

A retained root or unerupted tooth can cause pain under a denture. Radiographs will confirm the diagnosis.

Denture soreness with no apparent cause may be due to bruxism. This condition is characterized by highly polished occlusal facets. With these patients, explaining the problem and providing a generous free-way space may alleviate the condition.

Discomfort in specific regions of the mouth

As alveolar bone resorption progresses, bony ridges and prominences are liable to be accentuated. Examples of these are the mylohyoid ridge, the genial and mental tubercles, and the mental nerve in a superficial position.

These potential problems should have been diagnosed at the examination stage. Tin foil (0.3 mm) covering the appropriate areas of the working casts would have avoided this problem. If this has not been carried out, easing the corresponding area of the denture is a solution.

Surgery should be considered only as a last resort, after the dentures have been shown to be satisfactory.

If the mental nerve is subjected to pressure from the lower denture, paraesthesia (a burning or tingling sensation) of the lip of the same side may result. This is treated by adjusting the denture (Figure 25.1). Since the mental nerve runs forwards and downwards from the mental foramen, the lower denture should be eased in a forward and downward direction so as to clear the periphery.

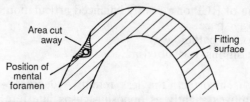

Figure 25.1 Area of denture eased for mental nerve pain

Loose dentures

There are four main causes:

1. Incorrect peripheral extension.
2. Incorrect position of teeth.
3. Unbalanced articulation.
4. Polished surfaces incorrectly shaped.

If the periphery of a denture is under-extended, a border seal cannot be effective. Correction can be made with a reline impression, following peripheral reconstruction of the base using greenstick impression compound.

Upper dentures are often insufficiently extended round the maxillary tuberosity into the pterygohamular notch (also called the pterygomaxillary fissure) (Figure 25.2).

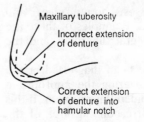

Figure 25.2 Upper denture: correct and incorrect extension round maxillary tuberosity.

Over-extension causes looseness particularly during speech. Disclosing wax helps indicate the specific region.

Aesthetic problems

Incorrect shade, shape or position of teeth are the prime causes of complaint. Theoretically if the patient is happy with the appearance of the teeth at the trial insertion stage, aesthetic problems should not occur.

Retching

This is usually triggered by contact of dentures with the palate or tongue. Ensuring that the thickness of the palate is not excessive is of help. Sometimes the palatal extension of the upper denture must be reduced until the patient no longer experiences this symptom. In severe cases exercises of brushing the palate with a toothbrush or deep breathing may help.

Masticatory inefficiency

In otherwise retentive and stable dentures, this may occur because of excessive free-way space or lack of balanced articulation. Very often this complaint comes from patients new to complete dentures who are expecting too much from them. Porcelain teeth probably provide the most efficient form of mastication, but are not widely used.

Cheek or lip biting

This can be remedied either by rounding sharp cusps and incisal edges, or increasing the buccal or labial overjet (Figure 25.3).

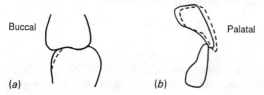

Figure 25.3 (*a*) Correct stoning of lower molar to prevent cheek biting; (*b*) resetting upper incisors to increase horizontal and vertical overlap prevents lip biting

Speech difficulties

Although these are common in the first few days after fitting dentures, long-term problems are rare. These can, however, be extremely difficult to treat (see Chapter 19, p. 141). The particular speech sounds which are causing difficulty should be identified and the corresponding area of the denture modified.

The dentures should be as stable and retentive as possible and the teeth should be in the neutral zone. The position of the upper molars and premolars is as important as the position of the anterior teeth. Moving teeth does not always help the problem.

Changing palatal contours may be beneficial with the incorpora-
tion of palatal rugae. Sometimes patients who suffer from
neuromuscular or cerebrovascular disease (including strokes)
blame speech problems on their dentures.

Food under dentures

This is a common complaint. Ironically, well fitting new dentures
seem particularly prone to suck debris under the fitting surface. If
the periphery of the denture is correctly extended and of the
correct width, the problem rarely occurs. Slight polishing of the
fitting surface sometimes helps. Some prosthetists believe the
accumulation of food under a denture is inevitable and tell their
patients so. Clearly the nature of the basal fit and ridge contour is
of fundamental importance.

Sore lips or tongue

This is not a common complaint. If the denture teeth are in the
correct position and no roughness is present on the polished
surface, it is possible such symptoms are caused by systemic
problems such as anaemia or, rarely, neoplasia.

Clicking teeth

This can occur if free-way space is insufficient or RCP is incorrect.
Porcelain teeth are more likely to cause this trouble during
mastication.

Summary

Remember that many of the foregoing problems can be
anticipated and hence avoided by a careful examination and
history procedure.

Berry (1985) believes that nearly all complaints with complete
dentures are due to one of three errors:

1. Excessive vertical dimension.
2. An interfering or locked occlusion.
3. Failure to reproduce exactly the features of a comfortable
   previous set of dentures.

Complaints of partial denture wearers

The problems encountered with partial dentures are very similar to those for complete dentures, and usually they can be solved in a similar manner. However, some problems are unique to partial dentures, and others require a different solution. These special problems are:

1. Looseness.
2. Inability to tolerate lingual bar or lingual plate.
3. Unsightly clasps.
4. Metallic taste.

Loose dentures

This can usually be remedied by providing sufficient clasps engaging suitable undercuts. However in many cases there are not suitable teeth available for clasping. In these situations several solutions may be possible:

1. Provision of multiple guide planes.
2. Creating undercuts with composite resins or providing contoured crowns.
3. Precision attachments.
4. Two-part dentures.
5. Interstitial retaining devices, e.g. ZA anchor.

In some patients it will become impossible to tighten a denture further. This must be explained.

Inability to tolerate a lingual bar or plate

This can be difficult to solve. Sometimes changing from a bar to a plate or vice versa satisfies the patient. If this is unsuccessful, buccal bars, continuous clasps, or precision attachments should be considered.

Unsightly clasps

This may be remedied by:

1. Placing the clasps more posteriorly.
2. Changing from occlusally to gingivally approaching clasps.
3. Removing the offending clasp altogether.
4. Using a ZA anchor or precision attachment.

Metallic taste

This is sometimes encountered with cobalt-chromium dentures soon after insertion and may be due to electrolytic action. Replacing amalgam restorations with non-metallic materials or gold alloys may be effective. If the taste persists and there is no likely systemic cause, the dentures may have to be remade in acrylic resin or gold alloy.

Chapter 26

Preprosthetic surgery

Preprosthetic surgery includes any surgical procedure carried out before the construction and insertion of a denture. It aims to improve denture support, stability, retention and comfort.

Preprosthetic surgery is elective, i.e. not strictly necessary. For example, a complete upper denture fractures frequently because of a large midline frenal notch. A simple frenectomy eliminates the need for the notch which is the primary cause of the fracture.

Preprosthetic surgery is divided into:

1. Hard tissue surgery.
2. Soft tissue surgery.

Hard tissue surgery

Excluding procedures carried out when inserting immediate dentures, hard tissue preprosthetic surgery includes the following procedures.

Removal of residual roots

These should be removed where they are causing symptoms, are associated with pathological change, or are in continuity with the oral cavity.

Modification of the alveolar ridge

An alveolectomy may be required when the shape of the ridge prevents the construction of a satisfactory denture as in the following conditions:

1. Irregular ridge shape.
2. Insufficient space for denture.
3. Undercut ridges.

Irregular ridge shape

This is often produced by the so-called socketed immediate replacement denture, particularly if it is worn for a long period after extractions. The ridge may be smoothed surgically to eliminate bony prominences which cause pain when in contact with the denture.

Irregular resorption will also result in unfavourable ridges which have been described as feather edge, knife edge, sharp or undercut. Patients with these conditions may benefit from surgical reduction and smoothing of the ridge, although in some patients those unfavourable contours may reform after surgery.

Insufficient space

Insufficient space for a denture is sometimes found between the maxillary tuberosity and retromolar pad. In such cases surgical reduction of the maxillary tuberosity may be performed.

Undercut ridges

Undercut ridges of great severity sometimes occur in the maxillary tuberosity and anterior labial areas.

Specific anatomical features

Specific anatomical features may become prominent following resorption and cause pain and discomfort under a denture. These include:

1. Genial tubercles.
2. Mental tubercles.
3. Mylohyoid ridges.
4. Palatal and mandibular tori.

Operative procedures to reduce or correct these have been described. Surgery is intended to improve the base extension and the quality of available supporting tissue.

Soft tissue surgery

Soft tissue preprosthetic surgery may include the following procedures.

Simple reduction

Simple reduction or elimination of frena, hyperplastic tissue or granulomas is usually simple and effective.

Removal of fibrous tuberosities

This is usually performed to create more inter-ridge space or to minimize a severe undercut.

Fibrous ridge

Reduction, modification or removal of fibrous tissue is sometimes performed surgically. Such surgery is done in an attempt to provide a more stable support for a denture. It is not always successful since a mobile fibrous ridge can be better than no ridge at all. Fibrous ridges are frequently seen at two sites: firstly, in the upper anterior region where the lower natural incisors and canines have been retained and adequate denture maintenance has not been carried out; and, secondly, in the lower anterior buccal sulcus where a denture flange has been able to induce a denture granuloma.

Sulcus deepening

Various operations have been described. Usually these procedures attempt to deepen the lower anterior labial sulcus, often using a mucosal or skin graft. There is evidence that in skilled hands they do produce a more stable denture.

Ridge augmentation techniques

See Chapter 24, p. 174.

Guidelines for preprosthetic surgery

The following is essential:

1. Full medical and dental history.
2. Radiographs.
3. Study casts before hard tissue surgery.
4. The elimination of all other causes of trouble with a denture. A competent prosthetist should confirm that the dentures are satisfactory with particular reference to RCP and base extension.
5. Respect for the patient's wishes. Preprosthetic surgery is elective.

The denture granuloma

This condition is usually seen as one or more rolls or flaps of fibrous tissue associated with the border of a denture flange. It is more commonly associated with a lower denture. It generally results from resorption of the alveolar ridge, allowing the denture flange to sink and so irritate the sulcus mucosa. A tissue hyperplasia results if the irritation is allowed to continue for many months. Treatment consists of:

1. Ruthlessly easing the offending flange; or
2. Leaving out denture.
3. If conditions resolve within a month, reline or remake denture.
4. If condition does not resolve, either the granuloma must be removed surgically, or its presence accepted and the denture built around it.

Chapter 27

Prosthetic care of the elderly and very young

The percentage of people living beyond 70 years has increased dramatically over the last 50 years. Although there are fewer complete denture wearers now than at any other time over the last 50 years, people are being rendered edentulous later in life. This could well mean that the proportion of elderly patients with complete denture problems will rise.

Changes that occur with advancing age

The following are some of the changes that occur with advancing age:

1. Protein cross-linkages form, resulting in complex giant molecules. This is probably the basic cause of ageing.
2. Decrease in peripheral blood flow.
3. Reduced immunity and capacity for repair.
4. Retardation of rate of cell division.
5. Degeneration of the nervous system.

Prosthetic care

Treatment planning must include consideration of chronological, biological and psychological age. If the existing dentures are in reasonably good condition, a denture copying technique will minimize changes and enable the patient to accommodate to new dentures more easily.

If the denture-bearing mucosa is inflamed or ulcerated, it should be allowed to recover before impressions are taken. This may be achieved by leaving out the dentures for a few days or using a tissue conditioning material.

Denture duplication

This is an extremely useful technique for certain circumstances. Wearing complete dentures is a skill that is learnt subconsciously over the years, the oral muscles learning how best to stabilize a particular shape of denture. There are recorded cases of husbands and wives sharing complete dentures, and this feat could only be accomplished with considerable muscular skill by one of the partners. When new dentures are provided, adaptation to them is much quicker if the shape is exactly the same as the previous set.

Those particularly benefiting from a duplication technique are:

1. Patients who have worn dentures successfully for many years.
2. Elderly patients whose powers of adaptation are slow.
3. Patients needing replacement of immediate complete dentures, where a precise copy of the position of the teeth is required.

Many techniques have been described for denture duplication. A simple method is described below.

1. One half of a denture duplicating flask is filled with alginate impression material and the denture pressed occlusal surface down onto the unset material.
2. When set, the exposed alginate is smeared with petroleum jelly.
3. The second half of the flask is filled with alginate impression material. This is then married up with the other half of the flask so that the denture is completely surrounded by impression material.
4. When the alginate has set, the two halves of the flask are separated and the denture removed.
5. Two sprue channels are cut into the alginate material so that self-curing acrylic resin can be run into the mould to fill the denture space.
6. Acrylic resin is run into the flask. When set the copy denture is removed and the sprues cut off.
7. The upper and lower dentures are mounted on an articulator. A wax wafer registration of jaw relationship may be taken before the duplication procedure if the occlusion is unclear, or if the vertical dimension is to be increased. It is used now if necessary.
8. The plastic teeth are cut off the duplicate denture and replaced with denture teeth, being fixed to the base with wax.
9. The dentures are tried in and corrections made as necessary. A reline impression is taken within the dentures. Note: Often the base extension is incorrect. Should one wish to correct it –

which is not always a wise thing with the elderly patient – it may be perfected with greenstick compound before the reline impression.

10. The dentures are processed in the usual manner.

Treatment of extreme resorption

The denture must utilize all the available supporting tissues. A broad anatomical base with narrow teeth is desirable. A generous free-way space will reduce the load applied to the ridge. Use of teeth with flatter cusps reduces horizontal displacing forces. Relief using 0.3 mm tin foil should be applied over prominent sharp ridges and over superficial mental foramina.

With diminished salivary flow, zinc oxide/eugenol impression paste may stick to the dry mucous membrane and burn more than usual. An elastomeric impression material should be used in these cases.

Denture labelling

In institutions or hospitals dentures are easily lost or interchanged. This can be prevented by using commercial denture marking kits or making small labels in the laboratory. These are inserted into the palatal or lingual surface of the denture and state the patient's name and sometimes other details such as hospital record number.

The non-ambulant geriatric patient

If a patient is bedridden, domiciliary visits can be made to construct new dentures or repair the existing set. For this purpose it is useful to have a kit of basic prosthetic instruments and materials which can be transported easily to the bedside. Even if bedridden, a patient's quality of life and pride in their appearance can be improved with adequate dentures.

Prosthetic appliances for children

Children may require partial – or occasionally – complete dentures. These are extremely well tolerated.

Problems associated with providing prostheses for children

1. The child is often wary or upset as extractions have often been performed at the previous visit.
2. The size of trays available for children is limited.
3. Recording jaw relationships may be difficult (but this does not seem to be critical with children).
4. Partial denture design. Small bulbous crowns may have insufficient undercuts. Adams cribs can sometimes be usefully used, particularly on permanent first molars.
5. Swallowing or inhalation of the appliance. The child should be told to take the appliance out for contact sports. The denture should be made radio-opaque with metal inserts or with special acrylic resin so that, should the denture be inhaled or swallowed, it can easily be located radiographically.
6. Teeth erupting beneath the denture. Frequent visits are required for removal of acrylic over erupting teeth. Caries prevention must be encouraged with dietary advice, oral hygiene instruction, fluoride gels, etc.
7. The need for frequent replacement dentures.

Chapter 28

Immediate complete dentures

General description

Immediate complete dentures are inserted at the same appointment as a dental clearance. In the earlier years of this century it was common practice to remove all standing teeth, often for patients in their early twenties, and insert immediate dentures.

Until the 1960s it was also accepted practice to leave a patient edentulous for 3–6 months after extractions, before constructing conventional complete dentures. This avoided the problems of ill-fitting dentures following the initial rapid resorption of the edentulous ridge.

The creeping denture

Fewer immediate complete dentures are now inserted and fewer teeth usually need to be removed before insertion. Since the trend is for patients to become edentulous much later in life, the transition to complete dentures can more easily be tolerated if it is a gradual process. This is achieved by initially constructing a partial denture – often in acrylic – and progressively extracting and adding teeth to it; hence the name *creeping denture*. The creeping denture is usually the best form of treatment for the elderly patient whose remaining natural teeth have a poor prognosis.

Advantages of immediate complete dentures

These are:

1. Aesthetics. Obviously most patients do not want to be seen without anterior teeth. Moreover, with immediate dentures the replacement artificial teeth can match their natural predecessors in position, shape and colour.
2. Correct positioning of teeth. The importance of placing all teeth within the neutral zone has been discussed earlier in this

book. This is easily accomplished with immediate complete dentures, as the artificial teeth may be set in the same position as their natural predecessors.

3. Better patient adaptability. Since the patients are wearing dentures immediately after extractions, they usually learn quickly to adapt to the new appliance. This is not the case if the patients are not provided with dentures for some months following a clearance.

4. Less alveolar bone resorption. Johnson (1964) has shown that maxillary bone resorption in patients provided with immediate complete dentures was less than in patients left edentulous and not fitted with dentures.

5. Less postoperative haemorrhage. Some clinicians believe that there is less postoperative bleeding with immediate dentures, as they act as a form of pressure pack.

Disadvantages of immediate complete dentures

1. Need for frequent adjustments. This is really the only disadvantage of immediate dentures. Since there is often a rapid change of alveolar ridge shape following extractions, immediate complete dentures quickly become ill-fitting. Relines usually solve this problem, but if loss of alveolar bone is severe, new dentures may be required.

Clinical procedures

The clinical procedures for immediate complete dentures are very similar to those for conventional complete dentures. However, there are three principal differences.:

1. The clinical stage of occlusal registration can often be omitted if there are sufficient opposing teeth to show PMI.

2. Some clinicians reduce the occlusal vertical dimension on the articulator by about 2 mm before processing (a procedure that is only accurate if a facebow recording has been used). This is because it has been shown that when a patient is rendered edentulous the vertical face height may decrease.

3. The trial insertion stage often cannot give a true picture of the aesthetics and occlusion, since there are still standing natural teeth around which the trial denture has to be inserted.

In summary, therefore, the usual clinical procedure for the production of immediate complete dentures is as follows:

1. Thorough clinical and radiological examination.
2. Decision that the best treatment is the extraction of the remaining teeth and provision of immediate dentures.
3. In complex cases the study casts should be mounted on a simple hinge articulator. This will aid the decision as to the number and order of teeth to be extracted, and will help in discussions with the patient.
4. Discussion with patient.
5. Primary impressions. Usually alginate in stock trays.
6. Secondary impressions. Usually taken in alginate in special trays, but elastomeric impression material may be used. This stage is often omitted in general dental practice.
7. Registration of RCP. If many opposing teeth are present this stage may be omitted since PMI can be obtained from the stone casts. (Note that with immediate complete dentures either RCP or PMI may be recorded according to the occlusion of the standing teeth.)
8. Trial insertion.
9. Insertion after extraction of remaining teeth.
10. Reviews and relining as necessary.

Advice to patients

The advice given to patients with immediate complete dentures is the same as for complete dentures (see p. 153) but with the following additional points:

1. Do not take your dentures out for the first 24 hours after they have been fitted. If they are removed you may not be able to get them back in.
2. If your mouth hurts after having your teeth extracted, take a pain killer such as soluble paracetamol in the dosage shown on the packet.

Review stages

After 24 hours the patient is reviewed. The surgeon should remove the dentures and inspect the mouth for areas of denture trauma; any necessary adjustments are carried out. Pressure-indicating paste is most valuable at this stage to show pressure areas.

If, at the 24 hour visit, the mouth is healing well and only minimal adjustments are required to the denture fitting surface and occlusion, the patient should be seen in a further six days; otherwise in two or three days.

One week after extractions the patient attends for a further review. If progress has been satisfactory, an appointment is made three months ahead to assess the necessity for relining the denture. If many teeth have been extracted a review in a further month may be considered desirable.

Relining immediate complete dentures

Because there is a rapid phase of alveolar bone resorption following extractions, immediate complete dentures can become very loose soon after insertion. The degree of alveolar bone loss following extractions will be dependent on the number of teeth removed and the physiology of the patient. Relining should not be done until three months have elapsed, since otherwise a second reline may be required within a further short space of time. Radiographic studies have shown that rapid resorption occurs for about six months following the extraction of teeth. If a patient is unable to cope with loose immediate dentures shortly after insertion, temporary reline materials are available for this purpose.

When relining immediate dentures it is particularly important to check that the dentures are occluding in RCP. The occlusion may be incorrect because either:

1. Rapid resorption – particularly of the mandible – has caused the dentures to sink and shift horizontally; or
2. The patient has adopted a postural occlusion, usually because of movement of one of the dentures.

If the occlusion is to be corrected, it is most easily carried out as follows. A reline impression is taken inside the dentures. When the impression material has set, a precentric registration is taken in wax or any other suitable material. The occlusion is then ground-in on an articulator before relining.

Open and closed face dentures

An immediate denture may be made with a labial flange (closed face) or without a labial flange (open face) according to circumstances. The primary indication for an open face denture is where there is a deep labial undercut into which it would be

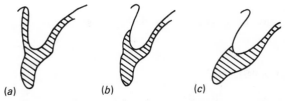

Figure 28.1 Sagittal section through maxilla to show ridge form associated with various types of flange: (*a*) closed flange; (*b*) semi-flange; (*c*) open flange

impossible to extend a flange (Figure 28.1). Surgery is often used to eradicate these undercuts (see Chapter 29), but some patients are unsuitable for surgery and others refuse it. Open faced dentures should only rarely be constructed for lower immediate complete dentures, since lower dentures with no flanges rarely have sufficient retention and stability. Some clinicians construct a flange extending half the length of a conventional flange and call this a semi-flange. This procedure makes the later construction of a full flange easier, when sufficient remodelling of the alveolus has caused undercuts to be abolished.

The flanged denture may be used with or without surgical trimming. If no trimming is performed the flange must be of thin section, otherwise undue prominence of the lip will result. Not infrequently the labial alveolar plate is so undercut that a decision must be made between an open faced denture or surgery.

When there is marked protrusion of the upper alveolar process, reshaping it can result in a better aesthetic appearance. This is particularly true if the patient has a short upper lip and shows the gingiva on smiling (i.e. has a horsey look). In such cases the appearance is improved by reducing the prominence of the labial alveolus, moving the upper incisors backwards, and raising the level of the gingival margin.

Advantages of open faced dentures

These are as follows:

1. No surgery required if severely undercut alveolar ridge present.
2. Better aesthetics possible if patient has high lip line.

Advantages of closed face dentures

These are as follows:

1. Better retention and stability, especially in lower jaw.

2. Relining easier.
3. Better protection of sockets, and probably assists in more rapid healing.

Laboratory procedures

Laboratory procedures are similar to those for complete dentures. The important difference is that the teeth must be removed from the stone cast and trimmed to the probable shape of the alveolus when the teeth have been extracted. This can only be done properly after a thorough clinical examination, involving measurement of pocket depth and often radiographs.

If a closed face denture is to be constructed the casts should normally be trimmed to a smooth rounded form along a line connecting the interdental papillae (Figure 28.2). With open face dentures the situation is different. The stone casts should be trimmed so that sockets are created which correspond to the depth of the periodontal pocket. This procedure improves the subsequent aesthetic appearance of the denture and often aids retention.

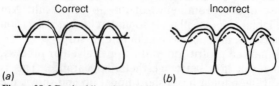

Correct   Incorrect

(a)   (b)

Figure 28.2 Dashed line shows (a) correct and (b) incorrect path of trimming stone casts for immediate dentures

It was formerly popular practice, especially with open face dentures, whatever the pocket depth, to trim the models so as to form sockets about 3 mm deep. This practice is often detrimental as it can leave the ridge irregular after healing, instead of smooth and rounded.

Clear acrylic templates
If alveolar surgery is planned prior to the insertion of immediate dentures, clear acrylic templates should be constructed. The degree of surgical remodelling planned can then be checked during the operation.

The surgeon himself must trim the stone casts. The final shape of the edentulous ridge must be based on a careful clinical examination.

The technician constructs the template by casting a duplicate of the trimmed model. An appropriate thickness of wax is then laid down. The template is then processed in self-curing acrylic resin, or heat-cured resin which is more transparent.

Full details of the techniques used to trim stone casts are given in Chapter 29.

Chapter 29

Surgical procedures for immediate dentures

Most surgical procedures performed prior to the insertion of immediate complete dentures are for the removal of deep bony undercuts, usually in the upper labial region. Removal of such undercuts means that a fully flanged denture can be inserted (Figure 29.1).

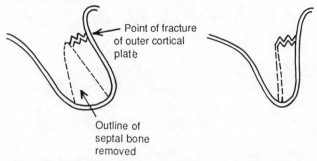

Figure 29.1 Maxilla in sagittal section before and after alveolectomy

Most patients requiring immediate dentures will not require any bone surgery. There are two principal techniques for remodelling labial alveolar bone, namely:

1. Septal alveolectomy.
2. Radical alveolectomy.

Septal alveolectomy

In this procedure the interdental septa are removed and the outer cortical plate rotated inwards. It is usually carried out in the region between the upper canines. The surgical procedure is as follows:

1. Extract anterior teeth.
2. Remove interdental septa with narrow tapering Rongeur forceps, or with a bur.

3. Make three vertical incisions in outer cortical plate by bringing fissure bur from socket outwards towards mucoperiosteum. These bony fissures should be in the midline and at the lateral border of the surgical area (i.e. usually the *3/3* sockets).
4. With the aid of a periosteal elevator lever the outer cortical plate outwards, which will fracture at its base. Then with finger and thumb press it inwards.
5. Check that bone recontouring is as planned with a clear acrylic template. If the template does not fit, or blanching of mucosa occurs, adjustments must be made – either by removing more bone or by adjusting the fitting surface of both template *and* immediate denture.
6. Trim any rough bony edges of the sockets with Rongeur forceps and the surplus gingiva with scissors.
7. Suture.

The cast modification prior to septal alveolectomy is:

1. Draw pencil line on cast along mucogingival margin.
2. Remove stone teeth.
3. Draw pencil line running through centre of sockets.
4. Remove stone between these two lines, rounding any sharp angles.

Radical alveolectomy

This procedure is used when gross recontouring of the alveolar bone is required (Figure 29.2) as follows:

1. Raise flap with a vertical incision in the mucosa in a region distal to the area of surgery, i.e. usually over the sockets of the first premolars.
2. Extract teeth.

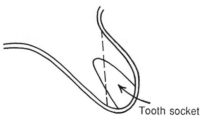

Tooth socket

Figure 29.2 Radical alveolectomy. Sagittal section of maxilla. Bone labial to broken line is removed

3. Remove as much of the outer cortical plate and interdental septa as required with burs, chisels or Rongeur forceps.
4. Check contouring with clear acrylic template. Adjust as necessary.
5. Suture.
6. Note: It is important to be judicious in one's trimming since the surgery will cause marked resorption. As a rule of thumb, if you are not sure whether you have trimmed sufficient bone – you have!

The cast modification prior to radical alveolectomy is:

1. Remove stone teeth.
2. Carve stone alveolar process until desired shape is produced. This will usually involve removing all, or most of the alveolar process.

Advantages of surgery for immediate complete dentures

1. Fully flanged dentures can be inserted affording better retention and stability.
2. Aesthetics can be improved. This is particularly the case in patients with a high lip line who show a lot of unsightly gum tissue.

Disadvantages of surgery for immediate complete dentures

1. Often associated with considerable postoperative pain and swelling.
2. Greater eventual loss of alveolar bone.

References and further reading

Anatomy

Last, R. J. (1984) *Anatomy. Regional and Applied,* 7th edn, J. and A. Churchill Ltd, London

Alveolar bone resorption

Dyer, M. R. Y. (1971) Alveolar bone resorption. *MSc Thesis,* Manchester University

Tallgren, A. (1972) The continuing reduction of the residual alveolar ridges in complete denture wearers: a mixed longitudinal study covering 25 years. *Journal of Prosthetic Dentistry,* **27**, 120

Watt, D. M. (1960) Morphological changes in the denture bearing area following the extraction of maxillary teeth. *PhD Thesis,* Edinburgh University

Jaw relationships

Basker, R. M., Davenport, J. C. and Tomlin, H. R. (1983) *Prosthetic Treatment of the Edentulous Patient,* 2nd edn, Macmillan, London

McMillan, D. R. and Imber, S. (1968) The accuracy of facial measurements using the Willis bite gauge. *Dental Practitioner,* **18**, 213

Dental materials

Coombe, E. C. (1986) *Notes on Dental Materials,* 5th edn, Churchill Livingstone, Edinburgh

Murray, I. D., McCabe, J. F. and Storer, R. (1986) The relationship between the abrasivity and cleaning power of the dentifrice-type cleaners. *British Dental Journal,* **161**, 205

Soft lining materials

Harrison, A. (1981) Temporary soft lining materials. *British Dental Journal,* **152**, 419

Treatment planning

Bremner, V. A. and Grant, A. A. (1971) A radiographic survey of edentulous mouths. *Australian Journal of Dentistry,* **16**, 17

Support of partial dentures

Watt, D. M., MacGregory, A. R., Geddes, M., Cockburn, A. and Boyd, J. L. (1958) Preliminary investigations of the support of partial dentures and its relationship to vertical loads. *Dental Practitioner,* **9**, 2

Partial denture design

Basker, R. M. and Davenport, J. C. (1978) A survey of partial denture design in general dental practice. *Journal of Oral Rehabilitation,* **5**, 215

Carlsson, G. E., Hedegard, B. and Kowuma, K. K. (1961) Studies in partial denture prosthesis. *Acta Odontologica Scandinavica,* **19**, 216

Christidou, L., Osbourne, J. and Chamberlain, J. B. (1973) The effects of partial denture design on the mobility of abutment teeth. An investigation. *British Dental Journal,* **135**, 9

Farrell, J. (1969) Partial denture tolerance. *Dental Practitioner,* **19**, 162

Plaque and partial dentures

Bates, J. F. and Addy, M. (1978) Partial dentures and plaque accumulation. *Journal of Dentistry,* **6**, 285

Bergman, B., Hugoson, A. and Olsson, C. E. (1977) Caries and periodontal status in patients fitted with removable partial dentures. *Journal of Clinical Periodontology,* **4**, 134

Brill, N., Tryde, G., Stoltze, K. and El Chamrawy, E. A. (1977) Ecologic changes in the oral cavity caused by removable partial dentures. *Journal of Prosthetic Dentistry,* **38**, 138

Precision attachments

Bolender, C. L. and Becker, C. M. (1981) Swinglock removable partial dentures: where and when. *Journal of Prosthetic Dentistry,* **45**, 4

Preiskel, H. W. (1985) *Precision Attachments in Dentistry,* 5th edn, Henry Kimpton, London

Plastic partial dentures

Dyer, M. R. Y. (1972) The Every type acrylic partial denture. *Dental Practitioner,* **22**, 243

Dyer, M. R. Y. (1984) The acrylic lower partial denture. *Dental Update,* 401

Every, R. G. (1949) Elimination of destructive forces in replacing teeth with partial dentures. *New Zealand Dental Journal,* **45**, 207

Resin retained bridges

Eshleman, J. R., Moon, P. C. and Barnes, R. F. (1984) Clinical evaluation of cast metal resin bonded anterior fixed partial dentures. *Journal of Prosthetic Dentistry,* **51**, 761

Gratton, D. R., Jordan, R. E. and Teteruck, W. R. (1983) Resin bonded bridges: the state of the art. *Ontario Dentist,* **5**, 217

Articulators

Craddock, F. W. (1949) Accuracy and practical value of records of condylar path inclination. *Journal of the American Dental Association,* **38**, 697

Watt, D. M. (1968) A study of the reproducibility of articulator settings from graphic records of mandibular movement. *Dental Practitioner,* **19**, 119

Masticatory performance of dentures

Brewer, A. A., Reibel, P. R. and Nassif, N. J. (1967) Comparison of zero degree teeth and anatomic teeth on complete dentures. *Journal of Prosthetic Dentistry,* **17**, 28

Kapur, K. K. and Soman, S. (1965) The effect of denture factors on masticatory performance. *Journal of Prosthetic Dentistry,* **15**, 662

Watt, D. M., MacGregory, A. R., Geddes, M., Cockburn, A. and Boyd, J. L. (1958) A preliminary investigation of the support of partial dentures and its relationship to vertical loads. *Dental Practitioner,* **9**, 2

Aesthetics

Mavroskoufis, F. and Ritchie, G. M. (1980) The face form as a guide for the selection of maxillary central incisors. *Journal of Prosthetic Dentistry,* **43**, 501

Phonetics
Lawson, W. A. and Bond, E. K. (1969) Speech and its relation to dentistry. *Dental Practitioner,* **19**, 150

Anthropoidal pouch
Matthews, E. W. (1964) The lower denture – the anthropoidal pouch technique. In *Principles of Full Denture Prosthesis,* 6th edn (ed. W. Fish), Staples Press, London, pp. 117–120

Denture stomatitis and related problems
Davenport, J. C. (1970) The oral distribution of *Candida* in denture stomatitis. *British Dental Journal,* **129**, 151
Basker, R. M., Sturdee, D. W. and Davenport, J. C. (1978) Patients with burning mouths. *British Dental Journal,* **145**, 9

Denture problems
Berry, D. C. (1985) Denture problems. *Annual Report of Medical Protection Society,* 1985

Implants
Branemark, P. I., Zarb, G. A. and Albrektsson, T. (1985) *Tissue Integrated Prosthesis: Osseointegration in Clinical Dentistry,* Quintessence Publishing, Chicago

Denture duplication and closed mouth impressions
Farrell, J. (1976) *Full Dentures. A Personal View,* Henry Kimpton, London

Preprosthetic surgery
Watson, C. J. (1987) Masticatory performance before and after mandibular vestibuloplasty. *British Dental Journal,* **162**, 417

Immediate dentures
Johnson, K. (1964) Study of the dimensional changes occurring in the maxilla after tooth extraction. *Australian Dental Journal,* **9**, 6
Nairn, R. I. and Cutress, T. W. (1967) Changes in mandibular position following removal of the remaining teeth, and insertion of immediate complete dentures. *Journal of Prosthetic Dentistry,* **44**, 595

Index